Metabolic-Associated Fatty Liver Disease

Editors

SHEROUK FOUDA
JOSEPH M. PAPPACHAN

ENDOCRINOLOGY AND METABOLISM CLINICS OF NORTH AMERICA

www.endo.theclinics.com

Consulting Editor
ROBERT RAPAPORT

September 2023 • Volume 52 • Number 3

ELSEVIER

1600 John F. Kennedy Boulevard ● Suite 1800 ● Philadelphia, Pennsylvania, 19103-2899

http://www.theclinics.com

ENDOCRINOLOGY AND METABOLISM CLINICS OF NORTH AMERICA Volume 52, Number 3
September 2023 ISSN 0889-8529, ISBN 13: 978-0-443-18407-9

Editor: Taylor Hayes
Developmental Editor: Jessica Cañaberal

Endocrinology and Metabolism Clinics of North America (ISSN 0889-8529) is published quarterly by Elsevier Inc., 360 Park Avenue South, New York, NY 10010-1710. Months of issue are March, June, September, and December. Periodicals postage paid at New York, NY and additional mailing offices. Subscription prices are USD 406.00 per year for US individuals, USD 907.00 per year for US institutions, USD 100.00 per year for US students and residents, USD 481.00 per year for Canadian individuals, USD 1121.00 per year for Canadian institutions, USD 527.00 per year for international individuals, USD 1121.00 per year for international institutions, USD 100.00 per year for Canadian students/residents, and USD 245.00 per year for international students/residents. To receive student/resident rate, orders must be accompanied by name of affiliated institution, date of term, and the signature of program/residency coordinator on institution letterhead. Orders will be billed at individual rate until proof of status is received. Foreign air speed delivery is included in all *Clinics* subscription prices. All prices are subject to change without notice. **POSTMASTER:** Send address changes to *Endocrinology and Metabolism Clinics of North America*, Elsevier Health Sciences Division, Subscription Customer Service, 3251 Riverport Lane, Maryland Heights, MO 63043. **Customer Service: Telephone: 1-800-654-2452** (U.S. and Canada); **1-314-447-8871** (outside U.S. and Canada). **Fax: 1-314-447-8029. E-mail: journalscustomerservice-usa@elsevier.com (for print support); journalsonlinesupport-usa@elsevier.com (for online support).**

Reprints. For copies of 100 or more, of articles in this publication, please contact the Commercial Rights Department, Elsevier Inc., 360 Park Avenue South, New York, NY 10010-1710; phone: +1-212-633-3874; fax: +1-212-633-3820; E-mail: reprints@elsevier.com.

Endocrinology and Metabolism Clinics of North America is covered in *MEDLINE/PubMed (Index Medicus), EMBASE/Excerpta Medica, Current Contents/Clinical Medicine, Current Contents/Life Sciences, Science Citation Index, ISI/BIOMED, BIOSIS,* and *Chemical Abstracts.*

Printed in the United States of America.

Contributors

CONSULTING EDITOR

ROBERT RAPAPORT, MD
Professor of Pediatrics, Emma Elizabeth Sullivan Professor of Pediatric Endocrinology and Diabetes, Icahn School of Medicine at Mount Sinai, Director, Emeritus, Division of Pediatric Endocrinology and Diabetes, Kravis Children's Hospital at Mount Sinai, New York, New York, USA

EDITORS

SHEROUK FOUDA, MSc, PhD
Doctor, School of Health and Biomedical Sciences, RMIT University, Melbourne, Victoria, Australia

JOSEPH M. PAPPACHAN, MD, FRCP
Professor, Department of Endocrinology and Metabolism, Lancashire Teaching Hospitals NHS Trust, Royal Preston Hospital, Preston, United Kingdom; Manchester Metropolitan University, Manchester, United Kingdom

AUTHORS

ANNA ALISI, PhD
Genetics of Complex Phenotypes Research Unit, Bambino Gesù Children's Hospital, IRCCS, Rome, Italy

SHIMA DOWLA ANWAR, MD, PhD
Department of Pediatrics, Boston Children Hospital, Harvard Medical School, Boston, Massachusetts, USA

AMBIKA ASHRAF, MD
Professor, Department of Pediatrics, The University of Alabama at Birmingham, Birmingham, Alabama, USA

TRIADA BALI, MD
Professor in Medicine-Hepatology, First Department of Internal Medicine, General Hospital of Athens "Laiko," Medical School of National and Kapodistrian University of Athens, Athens, Greece

THOMAS M. BARBER, MA (Hons Cantab), MBBS, DPhil (Oxon), FRCP, FHEA, FAoP
Doctor, Division of Biomedical Sciences, Warwick Medical School, Clinical Sciences Research Laboratories, University Hospitals Coventry and Warwickshire, Warwickshire Institute for the Study of Diabetes, Endocrinology and Metabolism, University Hospitals Coventry and Warwickshire, Coventry, United Kingdom

MARTIJN C.G.J. BROUWERS, MD, PhD
Division of Endocrinology and Metabolic Disease, Department of Internal Medicine, Maastricht University Medical Center, CARIM School for Cardiovascular Diseases, Maastricht University, Maastricht, the Netherlands

JAMES BROWN, FRCP(Edin), FRACP
Department of Thoracic Medicine, Cairns Hospital, Cairns, Queensland, Australia

EVANGELOS CHOLONGITAS, MD, PhD
Professor, Professor in Medicine-Hepatology, First Department of Internal Medicine, General Hospital of Athens "Laiko," Medical School of National and Kapodistrian University of Athens, Athens, Greece

LAMPROS CHRYSAVGIS, MD, PhDc
First Department of Internal Medicine, General Hospital of Athens "Laiko," Medical School of National and Kapodistrian University of Athens, Athens, Greece

MCCAWLEY CLARK-DICKSON, BMED, FRACP
Gastroenterology and Hepatology Fellow, Gastroenterology and Hepatology, Bankstown-Lidcombe Hospital, Bankstown, Australia

CHRISTY FOSTER, MD
The University of Alabama at Birmingham, Birmingham, Alabama, USA

SHEROUK FOUDA, MSc, PhD
Doctor, School of Health and Biomedical Sciences, RMIT University, Melbourne, Victoria, Australia

JACOB GEORGE, MBBS, PhD, FRACP
Robert W. Storr Chair, Professor of Gastroenterology and Hepatic Medicine, University of Sydney, Sydney, Australia; Head of Department, Gastroenterology and Hepatology, Westmead Hospital, Westmead, Australia

CAMERON GOFTON, BSCi, MBBS, MPH, FRACP
Director of Hepatology Services, Gastroenterology and Hepatology, Northern Sydney Local Health District, Head of Hepatology, Royal North Shore Hospital, St Leonards, Sydney, Australia; Hepatology Staff Specialist, Gastroenterology and Hepatology, Bankstown-Lidcombe Hospital, Bankstown, Australia

PETRA HANSON, MBChB, MRCP, FHEA, PhD
Doctor, Division of Biomedical Sciences, Warwick Medical School, Clinical Sciences Research Laboratories, University Hospitals Coventry and Warwickshire, Warwickshire Institute for the Study of Diabetes, Endocrinology and Metabolism, Coventry, United Kingdom

NISHA NIGIL HAROON, MD
Clinical Sciences Division, Northern Ontario School of Medicine, Health Sciences North Research Institute, Sudbury, Ontario, Canada

VENKATARAMAN JAYANTHI, MD, DM
Professor, Department of Hepatology, Sri Ramachandra Institute of Higher Education and Research, Chennai, India

MOHAMMED SADIQ JEEYAVUDEEN, MD, MRCP
Edinburgh Centre for Endocrinology and Diabetes, Royal Infirmary of Edinburgh, Edinburgh, United Kingdom

SANJAY KALRA, MD(Medicine), DM(Endocrinology)
Consultant Endocrinologist, Department of Endocrinology, Bharti Hospital, Past
President, Endocrine Society of India (ESI), Bharti Hospital and B.R.I.D.E, Karnal, India;
University Center for Research and Development, Chandigarh University, Chandigarh,
India; President Elect, South Asian Federation of Endocrine Societies (SAFES), India,
Board Member, International Society of Endocrinology (ISE), President, Indian
Professional Association for Transgender Health (IPATH)

NITIN KAPOOR, MD(Medicine), DM(Endocrinology), PhD(University of Melbourne)
Professor and Head(Unit 1), Department of Endocrinology, Diabetes and Metabolism,
Christian Medical College, Vellore, Tamil Nadu, India; Non-Communicable Disease Unit,
Baker Heart and Diabetes Institute, Melbourne, Victoria, Australia

CLAUDIA MANDATO, PhD, MD
Department of Medicine, Surgery and Dentistry "Scuola Medica Salernitana," University
of Salerno, Baronissi, Italy

ALEJANDRA MIJANGOS-TREJO, MD
Obesity and Digestive Disease Unit, Medica Sur Clinic and Foundation, Mexico City,
Mexico

ANOOP MOHAMED IQBAL, MD
Department of Pediatric Endocrinology, Marshfield Clinic Health Systems, Marshfield
Children's Hospital, Marshfield, Wisconsin, USA

MOHAMMAD NASSER KABBANY, MD
Cleveland Clinic Children's Department of Pediatric Gastroenterology Hepatology and
Nutrition, Cleveland, Ohio, USA

NADIA PANERA, PhD
Genetics of Complex Phenotypes Research Unit, Bambino Gesù Children's Hospital,
IRCCS, Rome, Italy

JOSEPH M. PAPPACHAN, MD, FRCP
Professor, Department of Endocrinology and Metabolism, Lancashire Teaching Hospitals
NHS Trust, Royal Preston Hospital, Preston, United Kingdom; Manchester Metropolitan
University, Manchester, United Kingdom

ANISH PRESHY, MBBS, MPHTM
Department of Medicine, Cairns Hospital, Cairns, Queensland, Australia

KADAKKAL RADHAKRISHNAN, MD
Cleveland Clinic Children's Department of Pediatric Gastroenterology Hepatology and
Nutrition, Cleveland, Ohio, USA

ZHEWEN REN, MS
Division of Endocrinology and Metabolic Disease, Department of Internal Medicine,
Maastricht University Medical Center, CARIM School for Cardiovascular Diseases,
Laboratory for Metabolism and Vascular Medicine, Maastricht University, Maastricht, the
Netherlands

COEN D.A. STEHOUWER, MD, PhD
Division of Endocrinology and Metabolic Disease, Department of Internal Medicine,
Maastricht University Medical Center, Maastricht, the Netherlands

NORBERTO CHÁVEZ TAPIA, MD, PhD
Obesity and Digestive Disease Unit, Medica Sur Clinic and Foundation, Mexico City, Mexico

MISAEL URIBE, MD, PhD
Obesity and Digestive Disease Unit, Medica Sur Clinic and Foundation, Mexico City, Mexico

KIRTHIKA VENKATESAN, MD, MPH
Caribbean Medical University School of Medicine, Willemstad, Curaçao; Walden University, Baltimore, Maryland, USA

CAROLYN VESPOLI, MD
Cleveland Clinic Children's Department of Pediatric Gastroenterology Hepatology and Nutrition, Cleveland, Ohio, USA

PAULINA VIDAL-CEVALLOS, MD
Obesity and Digestive Disease Unit, Medica Sur Clinic and Foundation, Mexico City, Mexico

MARTIN O. WEICKERT, MD, FRCP
Professor, Division of Biomedical Sciences, Warwick Medical School, Clinical Sciences Research Laboratories, University Hospitals Coventry and Warwickshire, Warwickshire Institute for the Study of Diabetes, Endocrinology and Metabolism, Centre of Applied Biological & Exercise Sciences, Faculty of Health & Life Sciences, Coventry University, Coventry, United Kingdom

ANKE WESSELIUS, PhD
Department of Epidemiology, NUTRIM School for Nutrition and Translational Research in Metabolism, Maastricht University, Maastricht, the Netherlands

Contents

Metabolic-associated fatty liver disease (MAFLD), formerly known as non-alcoholic fatty liver disease, is highly associated with the metabolic syndrome. Given its high heterogeneity in patients along with unpredictable clinical outcomes, MAFLD is difficult to diagnose and manage. MAFLD is associated with obesity, diabetes, metabolic derangements, lipid disorders, cardiovascular disorders, sleep apnea, sarcopenia, gut dysbiosis, and sex hormone-related disorders. Identification of risk factors is imperative in understanding disease heterogeneity and clinical presentation to reliably diagnose and manage patients. The complexity of MAFLD pathobiology is discussed in this review in relation to its association with common metabolic and nonmetabolic disorders.

Metabolic-associated fatty liver disease (MAFLD) has become the most common cause for chronic liver disease among children and adolescents globally. Although liver biopsy remains the gold standard for diagnosis, emerging technology, like velocity controlled transient elastography, a noninvasive method, is being utilized to evaluate degree of fibrosis in these patients. The discovery of multiple gene polymorphisms has brought new hope for possible treatment targets. However, this research is still ongoing, making lifestyle changes and weight reduction the current mainstay of treatment. This review briefly reviews the most recent data regarding the epidemiology, pathophysiology, diagnostic modalities, and treatment of pediatric MAFLD.

Since the nomenclature change from nonalcoholic fatty liver disease (NAFLD) to metabolic-associated fatty liver disease (MAFLD), much work has been undertaken to establish the clinical characteristics as well as the hepatic and extrahepatic complications of the different MAFLD subtypes. Currently, there has been significant work performed to evaluate previously acknowledged evidence in the lean NAFLD population to determine its applicability to the new entity. This article examines recently published data on lean MAFLD cohorts to highlight the prevalence, pathophysiological characteristics, associated liver fibrosis, genetics, hepatic and extrahepatic complications, prognosis, treatment, and research into this unique subtype of MAFLD.

Dyslipidemia has been linked metabolic-associated fatty liver disease (MAFLD). Several genes and transcription factors involved in lipid metabolism can increase susceptibility to MAFLD. Multiple parallel 'hits' have been proposed for developing hepatic steatosis, NASH, and MAFLD, including insulin resistance and subsequent free fatty acid excess, de novo lipogenesis, and excessive hepatic triglyceride and cholesterol deposition in the liver. This lead to defective beta-oxidation in the mitochondria and VLDL export and increased inflammation. Given the significant cardiovascular risk, dyslipidemia associated with MAFLD should be managed by lifestyle changes and lipid-lowering agents such as statins, fenofibrate, and omega-3 fatty acids, with judicious use of insulin-sensitizing agents, and adequate control of dysglycemia.

Both nonalcoholic fatty liver disease (NAFLD) and metabolic dysfunction-associated fatty liver disease (MAFLD) have been associated with incident cardiovascular disease (CVD), independent of confounders. Causality has recently been inferred by Mendelian randomization studies. Although these findings have contributed to current guidelines that recommend screening for and treatment of cardiovascular risk factors, it not yet clear how to position NAFLD/MAFLD in cardiovascular risk estimation scores and, consequently, which treatment targets should be used. This review aims to provide practical tools as well as suggestions for further research in order to effectively prevent CVD events in patients with NAFLD/MAFLD.

Metabolic-associated fatty liver disease (MAFLD) is the hepatic manifestation of metabolic syndrome and affects about 55% of people living with diabetes. MAFLD has been shown to be an individual risk factor for cardiovascular disease and its associated mortality. Although common, MAFLD is often underdiagnosed and not given adequate attention during clinical visits. This review highlights the most recent literature available on the evaluation and management of MAFLD in the presence of diabetes. The more recently available antidiabetic agents including glucagon-like peptide-1 analogs and sodium–glucose cotransporter-2 inhibitors have been shown to effectively manage both diabetes and MAFLD.

As an important sequela of the burgeoning global obesity problem, metabolic-associated fatty liver disease (MAFLD) has gained increasing prominence recently. The gut–liver axis (GLA) provides a direct conduit to the liver for the gut microbiota and their metabolic by-products (including secondary bile acids, ethanol, and trimethylamine). These GLA-related factors, including the host inflammatory response and integrity of the gut mucosal wall, likely contribute to the pathogenesis of MAFLD. Accordingly, these GLA-related factors are targets for possible preventive and treatment strategies for MAFLD, and include probiotics, prebiotics, bile acids, short-chain fatty acids, fecal microbiota transplantation, carbon nanoparticles, and bacteriophages.

The current evidence indicates a strong association between sarcopenia, the loss of muscle mass and strength, and metabolic-associated fatty liver disease (MAFLD). The two entities share many common pathophysiologic mechanisms, and their coexistence may result in higher rates of morbidity and mortality. Therefore, given their increasing incidence in the modern world, there is a need for a better understanding of the liver-muscle axis for early identification of sarcopenia in patients with MAFLD and vice versa. This review aims at presenting current data regarding the correlation between sarcopenia and MAFLD, the associated comorbidities, and the need for effective therapies.

Obesity is considered a twentieth-century epidemic and is a growing concern among health professionals. Obesity and its complications contribute to multiple chronic illnesses, such as type 2 diabetes (T2D), metabolic syndrome, obstructive sleep apnea (OSA), malignancy, and cardiovascular and liver diseases. In the last two decades, a bidirectional association between OSA and metabolic-associated fatty liver disease (MAFLD), independent of obesity, has been established. Both conditions have similar risk factors and metabolic comorbidities that may imply a common disease pathway. This review compiles the evidence and delineates the relationship between OSA and MAFLD from a clinical and diagnostic aspect.

Metabolic-associated fatty liver disease (MAFLD), the term proposed to substitute nonalcoholic fatty liver disease, comprises not only liver features but also potentially associated metabolic dysfunctions. Since experimental studies in mice and retrospective clinical studies in humans investigated the association between nonalcoholic fatty liver disease during pregnancy and the adverse clinical outcomes in mothers and offspring, it is plausible that MAFLD may cause similar or worse effects on mother and the offspring. Only a few studies have investigated the possible association of maternal MAFLD with more severe pregnancy-related complications. This article provides an overview of the evidence for this dangerous liaison.

Polycystic ovary syndrome (PCOS) affects around 10% of women in the reproductive age group and is characterized by ovulatory dysfunction, hyperandrogenism, and/or polycystic ovarian morphology. PCOS is highly associated with metabolic-associated fatty liver disease (MAFLD) as both diseases share common risk factors. At the time of diagnosis of PCOS, screening for MAFLD is necessary because most patients with MAFLD are asymptomatic. The importance of early detection of MAFLD in patients with PCOS is that a timely intervention in patients with steatosis or steatohepatitis can reduce the probability of liver disease progression.

Metabolic-associated fatty liver disease (MAFLD), previously known as nonalcoholic fatty liver disease (NAFLD), is the most common cause of liver disease in the world. Its prevalence is over 30% and is becoming the most common cause of liver transplants. Rates are rising along with obesity-related diseases. Risk factors for MAFLD include adverse lifestyles, genetic variations, advancing age, male sex, and alterations in the gut microbiota. Extrahepatic complications include cardiovascular disease, renal dysfunction, and colorectal cancer. As there are no currently approved medications for MAFLD, management mainly focuses on lifestyle modifications.

ENDOCRINOLOGY AND METABOLISM CLINICS OF NORTH AMERICA

SERIES OF RELATED INTEREST

Medical Clinics
https://www.medical.theclinics.com
Primary Care: Clinics in Office Practice
https://www.primarycare.theclinics.com/

VISIT THE CLINICS ONLINE!
Access your subscription at:
www.theclinics.com

ENDOCRINOLOGY AND
METABOLISM CLINICS OF
NORTH AMERICA

Foreword

Endocrinology and Fatty Liver Disease

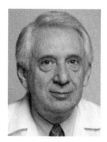

Robert Rapaport, MD
Consulting Editor

The last decade has witnessed a significant increase in the incidence and prevalence of obesity, diabetes, and their metabolic consequences in both the pediatric and the adult populations. Among those complications, there was a tremendous increase in what patients describe as fatty liver disease. Therefore, it is appropriate that an issue be devoted to metabolic-associated fatty liver disease. This issue discusses its pathogenesis and associated conditions, including its occurrence in the "lean" populations. Potential consequences and effects on metabolism and cardiovascular function are analyzed. Possible associations of fatty liver disease with the gut ok as is microbiome, sarcopenia, as well as with a prevalent condition of obstructive sleep apnea are discussed. In addition, pregnancy and polycystic ovarian disease association with fatty liver disease is examined. Last, current clinical practice recommendations about the management of fatty liver disease are addressed. I believe the contributions made in this issue will be welcomed by the Endocrinology Community.

Robert Rapaport, MD
Icahn School of Medicine at Mount Sinai
Division of Pediatric Endocrinology and Diabetes
Kravis Children's Hospital at Mount Sinai
New York, NY 10029, USA

E-mail address:
robert.rapaport@mountsinai.org

https://doi.org/10.1016/j.ecl.2023.04.001
0889-8529/23/© 2023 Published by Elsevier Inc.
endo.theclinics.com

Preface

Metabolic-Associated Fatty Liver Disease: A Disastrous Human Health Challenge

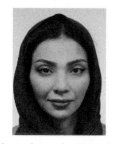
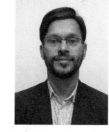

Sherouk Fouda, MSc, PhD   Joseph M. Pappachan, MD, FRCP
Editors

Metabolic-associated fatty liver disease (MAFLD) has emerged as the most challenging threat to human metabolic health in recent years, affecting about one-third of the global population.[1] While the disease is identified as the most common cause of liver failure in the world, the health consequences of MAFLD are much wider, involving almost every organ system in the body, further increasing the morbidity and mortality risk among sufferers. MAFLD is another silent killer, like hypertension and diabetes mellitus, as most patients with the disease are either asymptomatic or present with a nonspecific clinical picture, which is often missed by clinicians. Therefore, it is imperative to improve awareness among health care providers to ensure that patients are diagnosed and appropriately managed prior to the devastating complications of MAFLD settling in. Compiling 12 review articles by renowned authors from 9 different countries across 4 continents, we (the editors) attempt to provide the best evidence with expert guidance on this hot topic in this special issue of *Endocrinology and Metabolism Clinics of North America*.

We thank our peer reviewers, Dr Lakshmi Nagendra (Endocrinologist, Mysore, India), Professor Vekataman Jayanthi (Hepatologist, Chennai, India), Professor Anshu Gupta (Pediatric Endocrinologist, Virginia, USA), Professor Iskander Idris (Endocrinologist, Derby, UK), Professor Madhukar Mittal (Endocrinologist, Jodhpur, India), Dr Stergios Polizos (Endocrinologist, Athens, Greece), Dr Mohan Shenoy (Endocrinologist, Kerala, India), Dr Rahul Chaudhari (Hepatologist, Richmond, USA), Dr Sophie Willemse (Hepatologist, Amsterdam, Netherlands), Dr Shehla Shaikh (Endocrinologist, Mumbai, India), Professor Chan Wah Kheong (University of Malaysia), and Dr Stephen Vincent (Pulmonologist, Cairns, Australia) for their valuable contributions, which immensely helped to improve the quality of the articles published in the special issue. Last, but

Endocrinol Metab Clin N Am 52 (2023) xv–xvi
https://doi.org/10.1016/j.ecl.2023.03.001
0889-8529/23/© 2023 Published by Elsevier Inc.

endo.theclinics.com

not the least, we acknowledge the support from Jessica Nicole B. Cañaberal, Continuity Developmental Editor, *Endocrinology and Metabolism Clinics of North America*, Elsevier for her support at each stage of the editing process of this issue of *Endocrinology and Metabolism Clinics of North America*.

We admit that we were unable to compile literature exploring every aspect of MAFLD in this issue. However, we are sure the contributions by every author would enable physicians across the globe to provide the best care for patients with MAFLD. That is the best reward for us in editing this journal issue.

Sherouk Fouda, MSc, PhD
School of Health and Biomedical Sciences
RMIT University
Melbourne, Victoria VIC3001, Australia

Joseph M. Pappachan, MD, FRCP
Department of Endocrinology & Metabolism
Lancashire Teaching Hospitals
NHS Trust & Manchester Metropolitan University
Preston, PR2 9HT, UK

E-mail addresses:
sheroukf@gmail.com (S. Fouda)
drpappachan@yahoo.co.in (J.M. Pappachan)

*Corresponding author.

REFERENCES

1. Riazi K, Azhari H, Charette JH, et al. The prevalence and incidence of NAFLD worldwide: a systematic review and meta-analysis. Lancet Gastroenterol Hepatol 2022;7(9):851–61.

Pathobiology of Metabolic-Associated Fatty Liver Disease

Sherouk Fouda, MSc, PhD[a], Mohammed Sadiq Jeeyavudeen, MD, MRCP[b],
Joseph M. Pappachan, MD, FRCP[c,d,*], Venkataraman Jayanthi, MD, DM[e]

KEYWORDS

- Metabolic syndrome • Metabolic-associated fatty liver disease • Obesity
- Cardiovascular disease • Diabetes

KEY POINTS

- Metabolic-associated fatty liver disease (MAFLD) is a multisystem, multiorgan metabolic disorder although often clinically silent until complications develop.
- Associations of MAFLD include obesity, diabetes, metabolic syndrome, lipid disorders, cardiovascular disease, sleep apnea, sarcopenia, gut dysbiosis, and sex hormone disorders.
- Proper understanding of the pathobiology should enhance clinical care and development of therapeutic strategies.

INTRODUCTION

Metabolic-associated fatty liver disease (MAFLD) is becoming the most common chronic liver disease defined by the international consensus-driven panel of experts from 22 countries as the excessive accumulation of fat (>5%) in hepatic cells diagnosed histologically, imaging or increased specific blood biomarkers plus at least 1 of 3 metabolic criteria: overweight/obesity, established type 2 diabetes mellitus (T2DM) or the presence of at least 2 metabolic dysregulation factors (**Box 1**).[1,2] This so-called benign liver disease may progress from simple steatosis to the more serious

a School of Health and Biomedical Sciences, RMIT University, Melbourne, Victoria VIC3001, Australia; b Edinburgh Centre for Endocrinology & Diabetes, Royal Infirmary of Edinburgh, Edinburgh EH16 4 SA, UK; c Department of Endocrinology & Metabolism, Lancaster Teaching Hospitals NHS Trust, Royal Preston Hospital, Preston PR2 9HT, UK; d Manchester Metropolitan University, M15 6BH, UK; e Department of Hepatology, Sriramachandra Institute of Higher Education & Research, Chennai 600116, India
* Corresponding author. Department of Endocrinology & Metabolism, Lancaster Teaching Hospitals NHS Trust, Royal Preston Hospital, Preston PR2 9HT, UK.
E-mail address: drpappachan@yahoo.co.in

Endocrinol Metab Clin N Am 52 (2023) 405–416
https://doi.org/10.1016/j.ecl.2023.01.001
0889-8529/23/© 2023 Elsevier Inc. All rights reserved.

Box 1
Metabolic dysregulation

Definition of metabolic dysregulation in MAFLD

Any 2 of the 7 criteria mentioned below:
  WC ≥ 102/88 cm (Caucasian men and women) or ≥ 90/80 cm (Asian men and women)
  Prediabetes
  HOMA-IR score ≥ 2.5
  HDL cholesterol < 40 mg/dL (1.0 mmol/L) in men, < 50 mg/dL (1.3 mmol/L) in women
  Plasma triglycerides > 150 mg/dL (1.7 mmol/L)
  Blood pressure > 130/85 mm Hg hsCRP level > 2 mg/L

Abbreviations: HDL, high-density lipoprotein; HOMA-IR, homeostasis model assessment of insulin resistance; hsCRP, high-sensitivity C-reactive protein level; WC, waist circumference.[2]

---

nonalcoholic steatohepatitis (NASH), fibrosis, cirrhosis, and eventually may lead to hepatocellular carcinoma (HCC). The pathobiology of MAFLD remains unclear. However, the "multiple hit" theory is widely accepted highlighting the importance of various environmental and genetic factors playing a role in the pathogenesis of MAFLD.[3]

Metabolic derangements constitute the greatest risk factors for MAFLD due to their strong association with the metabolic syndrome (MetS). Obesity and diabetes are highly associated with MAFLD affecting between 70% and 90% of individuals diagnosed with these conditions.[4] Other associations include dyslipidemia, hypertension, cardiovascular disease (CVD), and isolated metabolic derangement without obesity. Nonmetabolic associations, such as gut dysbiosis, sarcopenia, sleep apnea, and sex hormone-related disorders to name a few, also play significant roles in the development and/or progression of MAFLD. The complexity of MAFLD is an evolving puzzle that scientifically suffers from chronologic mismatches between clinical and pathologic information, causing difficulty in creating models for drug discovery and screening to conceive ideal treatment options for patients.

Currently, there are multiple diagnostic tools that can be used individually or in combination to efficiently and effectively diagnose MAFLD patients. A liver biopsy is the gold standard for diagnosis of this clinical entity. However, due to its invasiveness, new methods have been developed and are currently used in clinics. The histopathological evaluation of a biopsy provides a strong insight into the steatosis pattern, lobular and portal inflammation, hepatocyte ballooning, fibrosis, and patterns of injury.[5] Biochemical tests in combination with imaging methods have proven ideal for detecting steatosis and liver "stiffness" at screening and for managing progression of disease but have yet to replace a liver biopsy.

MAFLD is difficult to identify due to its asymptomatic nature and is often diagnosed during routine imaging studies, such as an ultrasound study of the abdomen. This presents a major challenge to the practicing physicians who pay more attention to liver biochemistry, which often remains unchanged. The diagnosis is therefore made when the patients have progressed to more chronic stages of the disease. Currently, there is no specific treatment approved for MAFLD. At present, the recommendations are to treat the underlying symptoms, the associated comorbidities and thereby improve patient's quality of life. The lack of understanding about the pathobiology of the disease can affect both patients and clinicians and overall have a significant negative influence on treatment and management strategies. The aim of this article is to review the pathobiology of MAFLD focusing on its association with MetS and extrahepatic disorders.

PATHOBIOLOGY OF METABOLIC-ASSOCIATED FATTY LIVER DISEASE
Primary and Secondary Metabolic-Associated Fatty Liver Disease

Phenotypically, MAFLD exists as either a primary or a secondary disease entity. Primary MAFLD is highly associated with obesity and MetS, comprises of a cluster of disorders such as diabetes, dyslipidemia, insulin resistance (IR), and hypertension. In secondary MAFLD, there is an increased influx and accumulation of lipids within the liver due to extrahepatic causes such as viral infections, genetic disorders, drug-induced liver injury, endocrine disorders, or surgery. Due to limited data on the phenotypes of MAFLD, it is often difficult to distinguish between the 2 types.

Complexity and Heterogeneity

MAFLD is chiefly recognized by the accumulation of triglycerides in at least 5% of hepatocytes.[5] Patients with MAFLD frequently have other comorbidities that may exacerbate steatosis and vice versa. The high variability of MAFLD in its clinical presentation, as well as the heterogeneity in histology, makes this entity a highly complex disorder that clinicians should be aware of. They should also try to identify the risk factors in MAFLD. This would help in understanding the disease heterogeneity, its extrahepatic organ dysfunction, and the unpredictable nature of the disease.

Metabolic Syndrome

As obesity rates increase, the prevalence of the MetS increases in parallel.[6] A European study consisting of 10 cohorts (163,517 individuals) of metabolically healthy obese subjects showed a high association between obesity and the MetS.[7] The MetS is recognized as a cluster of metabolic disorders that includes visceral adiposity, dyslipidemia, IR, hyperglycemia, and hypertension. The coexistence of MAFLD with comorbidities and its effect on patient's prognosis is an increasing concern that requires a better level of understanding of its pathogenic processes. A large US study with a cohort of 11,674 individuals investigating the prevalence of MAFLD and the rate of advanced fibrosis among individuals with MetS showed that MAFLD prevalence was significantly increased ($\sim$40%) with advanced fibrosis almost doubled in the presence of MetS.[8]

Not all obese individuals have components of the MetS predisposing them to T2DM or CVD, and vice versa; also not all individuals with normal body mass index (BMI) have a favorable metabolic profile. Studies have reported lean patients with MAFLD suffer metabolic derangement, visceral adiposity, and dyslipidemia.[2,9] Lean MAFLD with a prevalence of 10% to 20%[10] have recently been categorized by Vilarinho and colleagues into 2 subtypes: type 1 that occurs in individuals with visceral adiposity and IR but normal BMI and type 2 that occurs in lean individuals with hepatic steatosis secondary to a known or unknown disease.[11,12]

RISK FACTORS FOR METABOLIC-ASSOCIATED FATTY LIVER DISEASE

The most common risk factors currently recognized for MAFLD are excessive fat/high caloric intake, sedentary lifestyle, genetics and epigenetics, drugs, viral infections, and diverse gut microbiota composition (**Fig. 1**). Genetics and epigenetics play a vital role in the development of MAFLD wherein first-degree relatives of patients with MAFLD can pose a higher risk of developing the disease compared with the general population.[5] Several genomic-based studies have identified numerous genetic polymorphisms associated with MAFLD development and progression.[13,14]

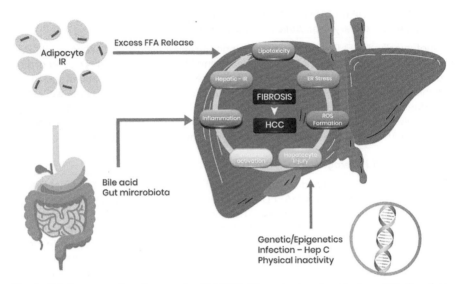

Fig. 1. Risk factors and pathogenesis of MAFLD. ER, endoplasmic reticulum; FFA, free fatty acid; HCC, hepatocellular carcinoma; IR, insulin resistance; ROS, reactive oxygen species.

DIETARY INTAKE

Diet plays a critical role in the pathobiology of MAFLD. A hypercaloric diet containing either excessive amounts of fats or carbohydrates is the main culprit in MAFLD. The large influx of lipids to the liver in the form of triglycerides resulting from a high fat diet, de novo lipogenesis or increased lipolysis of adipose tissue causes an imbalance in free fatty acid (FFA) input and output, with metabolic dysfunction and hepatic inflammation. Studies investigating the effects of excess caloric intake on liver fat accumulation in adults concluded that regardless of the macronutrient components, triglyceride accumulates in the liver rapidly, in as short as 3 days, with resultant IR and abnormal glucose metabolism in liver.[15]

Reduction in calorie intake, resulting in weight loss, has been shown to be a very effective therapy for overweight and obese patients with MAFLD. Clinical trials have shown substantial improvements in liver enzymes, liver steatosis, IR, and liver histology.[16,17]

SEDENTARY LIFESTYLE

A sedentary lifestyle is defined as low-energy expenditure due to insufficient levels of physical activity. Studies have shown a positive correlation between the prevalence of MAFLD and sedentary time after adjusting for most metabolic confounders.[18,19] An association between physical inactivity and unfavorable cardiometabolic and hepatic outcomes has been demonstrated. The beneficial effect of lifestyle intervention remains a critical component and first-line treatment of MAFLD.

VIRAL INFECTION AND GUT MICROBIOTA

Viral infections are recognized as a MAFLD risk factor due to their strong association with the development and progression of MAFLD. Acquired hepatotropic viruses such as hepatitis B and hepatitis C are known to cause liver inflammation and MAFLD progression to liver cirrhosis. Conversely, steatosis may cause an impairment in hepatic microbial clearance due to altered hepatic microcirculation thereby causing an enhanced susceptibility to fungal and bacterial infections.

The bidirectional relationship between the gut and the liver is referred to as the gut–liver axis. Recently, the gut–liver axis has been studied extensively in terms of gut microbiota alterations and MAFLD pathobiology. In fact, patients with MAFLD were found to exhibit gut dysbiosis with an imbalance between harmful and beneficial bacteria.[20] It is unclear whether dysbiosis is a direct cause of MAFLD or is involved in its pathogenesis. However, many preclinical and clinical studies suggest that gut microbiota dysbiosis acts as a key risk factor in the development of MAFLD.[20–22] Studies on microbiota signatures from patients with MAFLD have revealed that as the disease progresses, there is an increase in gram-negative bacteria and a decrease in gram-positive bacteria, with a shift from beneficial to harmful microbes.[20,22] Thus, the proinflammatory immune cells lead to the development of a metabolically toxic environment in the gut–liver axis.

CHILDHOOD AND ADOLESCENT ASSOCIATIONS

Pediatric MAFLD continues to be a topic that is underrecognized, understudied, and undermanaged to this date. Despite this, MAFLD has become the most prevalent chronic liver disease with a prevalence of 10% to 20% of the general pediatric population.[23] As seen with adult MAFLD, pediatric MAFLD is also strongly linked with metabolic risk factors such as visceral adiposity, dyslipidemia, IR, and CVD. Histologically, children have the same morphologic changes in the liver as is seen in adults while the patterns of fat accumulation and fibrotic lesions seem to differ between the 2 populations.[24]

CLINICAL ASSOCIATION OF METABOLIC-ASSOCIATED FATTY LIVER DISEASE WITH METABOLIC/NONMETABOLIC DISORDERS
Metabolic Diseases

Obesity and diabetes
Excess fat is stored ectopically in tissues such as muscle and liver where lipotoxicity can promote IR in these tissues with the development of MetS. Hepatic fat accumulation in MAFLD is mainly attributed to triglyceride content in the liver and is transported from the visceral adipose tissue. Excess circulating FFAs increase hepatic steatosis with the development of IR and eventually T2DM. The prevalence of MAFLD in obesity varies between 60% and 95%, whereas the prevalence of T2DM with MAFLD varies between 30% and 80%.[4] Visceral adipose tissue is known to be more metabolically active, compared with subcutaneous adipose tissue, which could induce metabolic stress, upregulation of proinflammatory signaling cascades, oxidative stress, cell injury, and death. This may trigger a systemic inflammatory response and increase peripheral IR by altered fat distribution and adipose tissue functionality.

IR can trigger lipolysis, increase the influx of FFAs to the liver and enhance hepatic de novo lipogenesis, adipokine, and inflammatory cytokine production. T2DM is considered a risk factor for the progression of MAFLD to NASH, cirrhosis, and HCC. The complexity in the pathobiology of the mutual interaction between T2DM and MAFLD deserves further research for impactful decision-making in public health and providing personalized treatment to reduce the risk of extrahepatic comorbidities and complications of MAFLD.

Metabolic derangement without obesity (lean metabolic-associated fatty liver disease)

Lipid derangement in lean individuals with MAFLD can be described as an increase in lipolysis and large release of adipokines causing an immense influx of FFA and accumulation in viscera, including the liver. Visceral adiposity without overweight is a key feature of "lean" MAFLD. The prevalence of MAFLD in lean individuals varies from 5% to 26%.[10] The differences are largely due to variations in the BMI cutoff that is used to classify individuals who are lean.[25] These individuals have distinct differences in metabolic, biochemical, and inflammatory changes compared with healthy subjects.[10] Moreover, they have a more favorable hepatic profile, which includes better histologic grading of steatohepatitis and fibrosis, compared with patients with obese MAFLD.[10] They have, however, similar characteristics of patients with obese MAFLD in terms of age, gender, and metabolic markers.[10,26] Interestingly, several meta-analyses on patients with MAFLD showed that patients with lean MAFLD have higher all-cause mortality and an increased risk of several extrahepatic events such as T2DM than patients with nonlean (obese) MAFLD.[10,27,28]

Nonmetabolic Diseases

Cardiovascular disease

MAFLD is considered a risk factor for CVD and is associated with other cardiovascular risk factors that include IR, dyslipidemia, and T2DM.[29,30] Hepatic steatosis has been shown to increase carotid atherosclerosis by modifying the carotid artery intimal thickness leading to carotid plaques.[31] Elevated biochemical markers such as γ-glutamyl transferase and alanine transaminase, in MAFLD patients with T2DM, can predict the presence of CVD.[32,33] Studies show that patients with MAFLD are likely to suffer from myocardial insults (ischemia/reperfusion injury/insult), abnormal left ventricular structure and diastolic dysfunction contributing to an increased risk of heart failure and cardiovascular mortality. Indeed, advanced MAFLD with liver injury is strongly associated with an atherogenic lipid profile, leading to alterations in triglyceride/high-density lipoprotein (HDL) cholesterol, total cholesterol/HDL, and low-density lipoprotein (LDL)/HDL ratios and an increased risk of IR.[34]

Sarcopenia

A decrease in muscle mass and/or strength, also known as sarcopenia, may exist with visceral adiposity causing a synergistic effect on health outcomes including metabolic disorders, cardiovascular events, and mortality. The combination of obesity and sarcopenia has been termed "sarcopenic obesity," which has been associated with high risk for CVD. A Korean sarcopenic obesity study has shown a close relationship between sarcopenic obesity with the MetS (Odds ratio 5.43) and arterial stiffness in 526 adults.[35] Recent studies have reported a relationship between sarcopenia and MAFLD where sarcopenia is a risk factor for the development and severity of MAFLD.[12,36] The prevalence of sarcopenia is also significantly increased in individuals with MAFLD and NASH and is associated with poor clinical outcomes such as severe hepatic fibrosis and increased mortality.[36] In another study, patients with MAFLD were at an increased risk of sarcopenia as indicated by the loss of skeletal muscle mass. This process was quicker in individuals with MAFLD compared with those without MAFLD.[37] Hence, sarcopenia and MAFLD share a cause–effect relationship that is complicated by IR in the background.

Sleep apnea

Obstructive sleep apnea (OSA) is recurrent obstruction of the upper airway during sleep leading to intermittent hypoxia. OSA is more common in obese individuals

(25%–35%) compared with the general population (1%–4%).[38] Increasing evidence suggests that OSA is part of the MetS and is considered a risk factor for MAFLD.[38,39] OSA is associated with IR and dyslipidemia; both components are linked to MAFLD. A reverse observation has also been reported.[39] Indeed, an increase in incidence of CVD with OSA can lead to MAFLD and even its progression. OSA is known to be individually associated with IR and T2DM, independent of obesity.[40] OSA was also found to be associated with inflammation activating major inflammatory mediators caused by hypoxia. This is amplified by the systemic inflammation resulting from obesity and MetS, which further increases IR and lipotoxicity.

Alterations in Female Hormones

Pregnancy

MAFLD in pregnancy have trebled during the past decade and is associated with adverse maternal and perinatal outcomes.[41] The potential implications of MAFLD for reproductive-aged women are increasing worldwide. Complications such as preterm birth, postpartum hemorrhage, hypertensive complications, elevated liver enzymes, and maternal or fetal death have been reported. Pregnancy by itself is an IR state and concomitant maternal obesity can further increase the risk for gestational diabetes, fatty liver, and hypertension.[41] The adverse risks of obesity and gestational diabetes on perinatal outcomes are well established, and therefore, clinical management of pregnant women with MAFLD is required to reduce maternal and perinatal morbidity and death.[42]

Polycystic ovarian syndrome

The close association between MAFLD and several endocrinopathies, such as hypothyroidism, polycystic ovarian syndrome (PCOS), hypopituitarism, growth hormone deficiency, hypogonadism, and hypercortisolism have been established in the literature. PCOS is an endocrine disease and thought to be part of the metabolic risk factor for MAFLD. Among the known causes of secondary MAFLD, PCOS, per se is a well-characterized risk factor and is an important cause of anovulatory infertility (10%) of women of reproductive age.[43] PCOS characterized by hyperandrogenism, is highly associated with risk factors for CVD, obesity (60%), MAFLD (50%), and IR (70%).[43] Many cohort studies have demonstrated that women with PCOS had a higher prevalence of MetS, MAFLD (35%–70%), and higher risk of IR regardless of BMI. A large meta-analysis of 17 observational studies, which included both women with PCOS and healthy women of matched age and BMI, concluded that women with PCOS had twice the risk of having MAFLD than healthy women.[44] Another pathobiological mechanism between MAFLD and PCOS is the likelihood of the downregulation of the LDL-receptor gene transcription, prolonging the half-life of very low-density lipoproteins and LDL, thereby causing the accumulation of fat in the liver, triggering MAFLD.[45]

Male hormonal disorders

Secondary hypogonadism refers to the inability of the hypothalamus or pituitary gland to produce enough follicle-stimulating hormone (FSH) and luteinizing hormone (LH) and is characterized by low concentrations of sex hormones, LH, and FSH. Male obesity-related secondary hypogonadism (MOSH) causes impairment in fertility, sexual function, bone mineralization, and fat metabolism.[46] Recent studies have reported a strong bidirectional association between MAFLD and MOSH. Low levels of testosterone are known to cause accumulation of abdominal fat with higher visceral adiposity compared with their healthy peers.[47] A significant proportion of men with MetS have low testosterone levels compared with healthy controls.[47] This explains

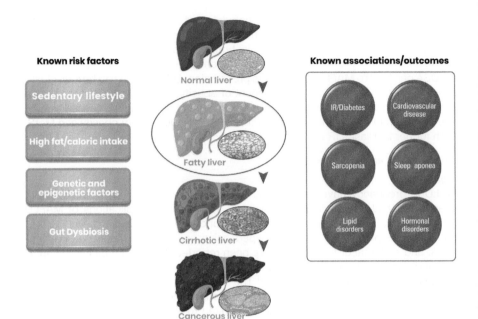

Fig. 2. MAFLD pathobiology. Risk factors associated with MAFLD, hepatic outcomes, and extrahepatic outcomes/associations, which may also contribute to fatty liver and vice versa. IR, insulin resistance.

why individuals with hepatic steatosis are more likely to have low testosterone levels. Clinical and experimental interventional studies that focused on testosterone replacement therapy showed an improvement in insulin sensitivity, BMI, liver fat content, and the hepatic steatosis.[48,49] The pathobiological mechanisms and associations of MAFLD are depicted in **Fig. 2**.

Clinical challenges/emerging concepts

Because there is no approved pharmacotherapy for MAFLD, research should focus on the development of new therapeutic strategies. In a recent study on subcutaneous semaglutide, 0.4 mg daily,[50] there was a significant resolution of NASH. This observation may enhance trials for newer drug molecules. The promising role of bariatric surgery needs more studies before formal clinical practice recommendations can be made. Emerging therapies for gut dysbiosis are the other areas of development for the future.

SUMMARY

The continuous effort in identifying risk factors for MAFLD may help in understanding disease heterogeneity and organ dysfunction to better improve patient outcomes and aid clinicians in disease management. The association of metabolic and nonmetabolic disorders with MAFLD can lead to hepatic and extrahepatic complications and further disease progression. Early diagnosis is key to better prognosis outcomes. Increasing disease awareness and finding innovative treatment strategies by including the use of metabolic and genetic profiles will help develop a better understanding of the pathobiology of MAFLD and create room for personalized medicine approaches. Therefore, impactful research to identify and classify MAFLD risk factors is a priority to understand relative contribution of components of MetS to the total burden and further improve failures at therapeutic trials to pave way to cost-effective health-care systems.

CLINICS CARE POINTS

- The heterogeneity in MAFLD is a result of its complex pathobiology.
- MAFLD is highly associated with the MetS.
- Identifying risk factors for MAFLD can improve patients' clinical outcome.
- Metabolic disease associations with MAFLD include obesity, diabetes, and dyslipidemia.
- Nonmetabolic disease associations with MAFLD include CVD, sarcopenia, sleep apnea, and male/female hormonal disorders.
- Immediate clinical implications of MAFLD vary among individuals.
- MAFLD poses major clinical and therapeutic challenges despite clinicians seeking to deliver the best possible patient care.

REFERENCES

1. Eslam M, Newsome PN, Sarin SK, et al. A new definition for metabolic dysfunction-associated fatty liver disease: An international expert consensus statement. J Hepatol 2020;73(1):202–9.
2. Godoy-Matos AF, Silva Júnior WS, Valerio CM. NAFLD as a continuum: from obesity to metabolic syndrome and diabetes. Diabetol Metab Syndr 2020;12:60.
3. Buzzetti E, Pinzani M, Tsochatzis EA. The multiple-hit pathogenesis of non-alcoholic fatty liver disease (NAFLD). Metabolism 2016;65(8):1038–48.
4. Dai W, Ye L, Liu A, et al. Prevalence of nonalcoholic fatty liver disease in patients with type 2 diabetes mellitus: A meta-analysis. Medicine (Baltim) 2017;96(39): e8179.
5. Younossi Z, Anstee QM, Marietti M, et al. Global burden of NAFLD and NASH: trends, predictions, risk factors and prevention. Nat Rev Gastroenterol Hepatol 2018;15(1):11–20.
6. Le MH, Devaki P, Ha NB, et al. Prevalence of non-alcoholic fatty liver disease and risk factors for advanced fibrosis and mortality in the United States. PLoS One 2017;12(3):e0173499.
7. van Vliet-Ostaptchouk JV, Nuotio ML, Slagter SN, et al. The prevalence of metabolic syndrome and metabolically healthy obesity in Europe: a collaborative analysis of ten large cohort studies. BMC Endocr Disord 2014;14:9.
8. Jinjuvadia R, Antaki F, Lohia P, et al. The Association Between Nonalcoholic Fatty Liver Disease and Metabolic Abnormalities in The United States Population. J Clin Gastroenterol 2017;51(2):160–6. https://doi.org/10.1097/mcg.0000000000000666.
9. Bhargav V, Jain M, Alen T, et al. Clusters and components of metabolic syndrome (MeS) as a predictor for fatty liver: A cross-sectional study. Journal of Diabetology 2021;12(4):434–41.
10. Young S, Tariq R, Provenza J, et al. Prevalence and profile of nonalcoholic fatty liver disease in lean adults: systematic review and Meta-Analysis. Hepatology communications 2020;4(7):953–72.
11. Vilarinho S, Ajmera V, Zheng M, et al. Emerging role of genomic analysis in clinical evaluation of lean individuals with NAFLD. Hepatol 2021;74(4):2241–50.

12. Kim Y, Han E, Lee JS, et al. Cardiovascular risk is elevated in lean subjects with nonalcoholic fatty liver disease. Gut and liver 2022;16(2):290.

13. Botello-Manilla AE, Chávez-Tapia NC, Uribe M, et al. Genetics and epigenetics purpose in nonalcoholic fatty liver disease. Expert Rev Gastroenterol Hepatol 2020;14(8):733–48.

14. Arrese M, Arab JP, Barrera F, et al. Insights into Nonalcoholic Fatty-Liver Disease Heterogeneity. Semin Liver Dis 2021;41(4):421–34.

15. van der Meer RW, Hammer S, Lamb HJ, et al. Effects of short-term high-fat, high-energy diet on hepatic and myocardial triglyceride content in healthy men. J Clin Endocrinol Metab 2008;93(7):2702–8.

16. Romero-Gómez M, Zelber-Sagi S, Trenell M. Treatment of NAFLD with diet, physical activity and exercise. Journal of hepatology 2017;67(4):829–46.

17. Wong VW-S, Wong GL-H, Chan RS-M, et al. Beneficial effects of lifestyle intervention in non-obese patients with non-alcoholic fatty liver disease. Journal of hepatology 2018;69(6):1349–56.

18. Ma Q, Ye J, Shao C, et al. Metabolic benefits of changing sedentary lifestyles in nonalcoholic fatty liver disease: a meta-analysis of randomized controlled trials. Ther Adv Endocrinol Metab 2022;13. 20420188221122426.

19. Wei H, Qu H, Wang H, et al. Associations between sitting time and non-alcoholic fatty liver diseases in Chinese male workers: a cross-sectional study. BMJ Open 2016;6(9):e011939.

20. Aron-Wisnewsky J, Vigliotti C, Witjes J, et al. Gut microbiota and human NAFLD: disentangling microbial signatures from metabolic disorders. Nat Rev Gastroenterol Hepatol 2020;17(5):279–97.

21. Fajstova A, Galanova N, Coufal S, et al. Diet rich in simple sugars promotes pro-inflammatory response via gut microbiota alteration and TLR4 signaling. Cells 2020;9(12):2701.

22. Loomba R, Seguritan V, Li W, et al. Gut microbiome-based metagenomic signature for non-invasive detection of advanced fibrosis in human nonalcoholic fatty liver disease. Cell Metabol 2017;25(5):1054–62.e5.

23. Berardis S, Sokal E. Pediatric non-alcoholic fatty liver disease: an increasing public health issue. Eur J Pediatr 2014;173(2):131–9.

24. Kleiner DE, Makhlouf HR. Histology of Nonalcoholic Fatty Liver Disease and Nonalcoholic Steatohepatitis in Adults and Children. Clin Liver Dis 2016;20(2):293–312.

25. Nishioji K, Sumida Y, Kamaguchi M, et al. Prevalence of and risk factors for non-alcoholic fatty liver disease in a non-obese Japanese population, 2011–2012. J Gastroenterol 2015;50(1):95–108.

26. Eslam M, El-Serag HB, Francque S, et al. Metabolic (dysfunction)-associated fatty liver disease in individuals of normal weight. Nat Rev Gastroenterol Hepatol 2022;19(10):638–51.

27. Ye Q, Zou B, Yeo YH, et al. Global prevalence, incidence, and outcomes of non-obese or lean non-alcoholic fatty liver disease: a systematic review and meta-analysis. Lancet Gastroenterol Hepatol 2020;5(8):739–52.

28. Tang A, Ng CH, Phang PH, et al. Comparative Burden of Metabolic Dysfunction in Lean NAFLD vs. Non-Lean NAFLD-A Systematic Review and Meta-Analysis. Clin Gastroenterol Hepatol 2022;S1542-3565(22):00669–73.

29. Targher G, Byrne CD, Lonardo A, et al. Non-alcoholic fatty liver disease and risk of incident cardiovascular disease: a meta-analysis. Journal of hepatology 2016;65(3):589–600.

30. Zeb I, Li D, Budoff MJ, et al. Nonalcoholic fatty liver disease and incident cardiac events: the multi-ethnic study of atherosclerosis. J Am Coll Cardiol 2016;67(16): 1965–6.
31. Sookoian S, Pirola CJ. Non-alcoholic fatty liver disease is strongly associated with carotid atherosclerosis: A systematic review. J Hepatol 2008;49(4):600–7.
32. Mantovani A, Mingolla L, Rigolon R, et al. Nonalcoholic fatty liver disease is independently associated with an increased incidence of cardiovascular disease in adult patients with type 1 diabetes. Int J Cardiol 2016;225:387–91.
33. Targher G, Valbusa F, Bonapace S, et al. Non-alcoholic fatty liver disease is associated with an increased incidence of atrial fibrillation in patients with type 2 diabetes. PLoS One 2013;8(2):e57183.
34. Arai T, Atsukawa M, Tsubota A, et al. Liver fibrosis is associated with carotid atherosclerosis in patients with liver biopsy-proven nonalcoholic fatty liver disease. Sci Rep 2021;11(1):15938.
35. Kim TN, Park MS, Lim KI, et al. Skeletal muscle mass to visceral fat area ratio is associated with metabolic syndrome and arterial stiffness: The Korean Sarcopenic Obesity Study (KSOS). Diabetes Res Clin Pract 2011;93(2):285–91.
36. Wijarnpreecha K, Kim D, Raymond P, et al. Associations between sarcopenia and nonalcoholic fatty liver disease and advanced fibrosis in the USA. Eur J Gastroenterol Hepatol 2019;31(9):1121–8.
37. Sinn DH, Kang D, Kang M, et al. Nonalcoholic fatty liver disease and accelerated loss of skeletal muscle mass: A longitudinal cohort study. Hepatology 2022;76(6): 1746–54.
38. Umbro I, Fabiani V, Fabiani M, et al. Association between non-alcoholic fatty liver disease and obstructive sleep apnea. World J Gastroenterol 2020;26(20): 2669–81.
39. Chung GE, Cho EJ, Yoo J-J, et al. Nonalcoholic fatty liver disease is associated with the development of obstructive sleep apnea. Sci Rep 2021;11(1):13473.
40. Vacelet L, Hupin D, Pichot V, et al. Insulin Resistance and Type 2 Diabetes in Asymptomatic Obstructive Sleep Apnea: Results of the PROOF Cohort Study After 7 Years of Follow-Up. Front Physiol 2021;12:650758.
41. Sarkar M, Grab J, Dodge JL, et al. Non-alcoholic fatty liver disease in pregnancy is associated with adverse maternal and perinatal outcomes. J Hepatol 2020; 73(3):516–22.
42. Hagström H, Höijer J, Ludvigsson JF, et al. Adverse outcomes of pregnancy in women with non-alcoholic fatty liver disease. Liver Int 2016;36(2):268–74.
43. Lonardo A, Mantovani A, Lugari S, et al. NAFLD in some common endocrine diseases: prevalence, pathophysiology, and principles of diagnosis and management. Int J Mol Sci 2019;20(11):2841.
44. Wu J, Yao X-Y, Shi R-X, et al. A potential link between polycystic ovary syndrome and non-alcoholic fatty liver disease: an update meta-analysis. Reprod Health 2018;15(1):1–9.
45. Baranova A, Tran TP, Afendy A, et al. Molecular signature of adipose tissue in patients with both non-alcoholic fatty liver disease (NAFLD) and polycystic ovarian syndrome (PCOS). J Transl Med 2013;11(1):1–8.
46. De Lorenzo A, Noce A, Moriconi E, et al. MOSH Syndrome (Male Obesity Secondary Hypogonadism): Clinical Assessment and Possible Therapeutic Approaches. Nutrients 2018;10(4):474.
47. Kapoor D, Aldred H, Clark S, et al. Clinical and biochemical assessment of hypogonadism in men with type 2 diabetes: correlations with bioavailable testosterone and visceral adiposity. Diabetes Care 2007;30(4):911–7.

48. Kalinchenko SY, Tishova YA, Mskhalaya GJ, et al. Effects of testosterone supplementation on markers of the metabolic syndrome and inflammation in hypogonadal men with the metabolic syndrome: the double-blinded placebo-controlled Moscow study. Clinical endocrinology 2010;73(5):602–12.
49. Nikolaenko L, Jia Y, Wang C, et al. Testosterone replacement ameliorates nonalcoholic fatty liver disease in castrated male rats. Endocrinology 2014;155(2): 417–28.
50. Newsome PN, Buchholtz K, Cusi K, et al. A Placebo-Controlled Trial of Subcutaneous Semaglutide in Nonalcoholic Steatohepatitis. N Engl J Med 2021; 384(12):1113–24.

Metabolic-Associated Fatty Liver Disease in Childhood and Adolescence

Carolyn Vespoli, MD[a],*, Anoop Mohamed Iqbal, MD[b],
Mohammad Nasser Kabbany, MD[a],
Kadakkal Radhakrishnan, MD[a]

KEYWORDS

- Fatty liver • Nonalcoholic fatty liver disease • Nonalcoholic steatohepatitis
- Metabolic-associated fatty liver disease • Metabolic syndrome

KEY POINTS

- Metabolic-associated fatty liver disease (MAFLD) has emerged as the most common cause of chronic liver disease among children and adolescents.
- Type I pediatric nonalcoholic steatohepatitis (NASH) shows a similar histopathologic pattern as adult NASH. However, type II pediatric NASH is different from type I NASH as well as adult NASH in that it is defined as the presence of steatosis along with portal inflammation and/or fibrosis in the absence of ballooning degeneration and perisinusoidal fibrosis.
- There are several single-nucleotide gene polymorphisms (*PNPLA3*, *TM6SF2*, *MBOAT7*, and *GPR120*) that are being studied as possible contributors to development of MAFLD and progression to NASH.
- The cornerstone of treatment of pediatric MAFLD is dietary improvement and increased physical activity.
- There are several emerging therapies that target various steps in the pathogenesis and progression of MAFLD in children that show promise for possible pharmacologic treatment options in the future.

INTRODUCTION

Metabolic-associated fatty liver disease (MAFLD), a recently proposed name change from nonalcoholic fatty liver disease (NAFLD) to encompass its close association with

---

[a] Cleveland Clinic Children's Department of Pediatric Gastroenterology Hepatology and Nutrition, 8950 Euclid Avenue, R Building, Cleveland, OH 44195, USA; [b] Department of Pediatric Endocrinology, Marshfield Clinic Health Systems, Marshfield Children's Hospital, 3rd Floor, 3D, 1000 North Oak Avenue, Marshfield, WI 54449, USA
* Corresponding author.
E-mail address: vespolc2@ccf.org

Endocrinol Metab Clin N Am 52 (2023) 417–430
https://doi.org/10.1016/j.ecl.2023.02.001
0889-8529/23/© 2023 Elsevier Inc. All rights reserved.

metabolic syndrome, has become one of the major causes for chronic liver disease among children and adolescents globally in the past few decades owing to the increasing prevalence of obesity in these age groups.[1] According to the World Health Organization, 39 million children under the age of 5 years were overweight or obese in 2020 and more than 340 million children and adolescents aged 5 to 19 years were overweight or obese in the year 2016.[2] According to the most recent data, the prevalence of childhood obesity-related MAFLD is found to be 52.1%, 39.7%, and 23.0% in Asia, South America, and Europe, respectively.[3] The obesity pandemic is still hitting the global population with the force of an approaching tsunami, which is expected to further worsen the prevalence of MAFLD and liver-related morbidity and mortality in the coming years in young adults. MAFLD is often associated with other diseases, such as hypertension, dyslipidemia, type 2 diabetes mellitus, gallstones, gastroesophageal reflux disease, obstructive sleep apnea, and depression, which substantially increase morbidity among the sufferers.[4] This evidence-based review provides the health care providers with the most up-to-date information on the pathophysiology, clinical evaluation, diagnostic approach, and management of MAFLD among children and adolescents.

EPIDEMIOLOGIC BURDEN

The global level prevalence of MAFLD increased from 19.34 million in 1990 to 29.49 million in 2017 among children and adolescents. The largest increase had been observed in the Middle East and North Africa.[1] MAFLD has emerged as the most common cause of chronic liver disease among children and adolescents. Based on a systematic review, prevalence of MAFLD in children in the general population is likely between 5.5% and 10.3%.[5] This wide range is likely due to regional differences, number of studies, cohort size, and diagnostic modality used. **Fig. 1** shows the estimated prevalence of pediatric MAFLD in every continent based on most recent data. **Fig. 2** shows the estimated prevalence among the obese, pediatric population.

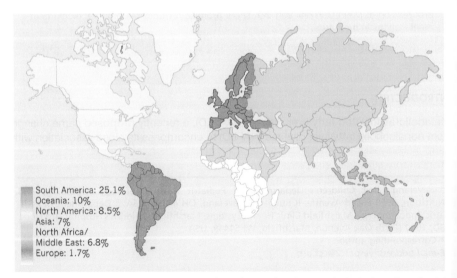

South America: 25.1%
Oceania: 10%
North America: 8.5%
Asia: 7%
North Africa/
Middle East: 6.8%
Europe: 1.7%

Fig. 1. Estimated MAFLD prevalence within the pediatric population. (Reprinted with permission, Cleveland Clinic Foundation ©2023. All Rights Reserved.)

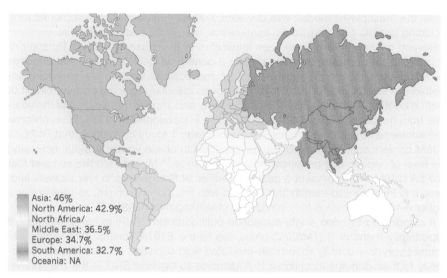

Fig. 2. Estimated MAFLD prevalence within obese pediatric population. (Reprinted with permission, Cleveland Clinic Foundation ©2023. All Rights Reserved.)

Asia: 46%
North America: 42.9%
North Africa/
Middle East: 36.5%
Europe: 34.7%
South America: 32.7%
Oceania: NA

MAFLD is considered one of the most common indications for liver transplantation in US adults.[5] Children with MAFLD are at increased risk of developing progressive liver disease.[6] Based on adult data, the annual burden associated with all MAFLD cases in the United States has been estimated at $103 billion, and projections suggest that the expected 10-year burden of MAFLD may increase to $1.005 trillion.[7] Based on a large population-based study, the mean cost per chronic liver disease–related hospitalization was $16,271, whereas the total national estimated cost for chronic liver disease–related hospitalizations from 2012 to 2016 was $81.1 billion.[8]

CAUSE

Similar to adults, MAFLD in children and adolescents includes a spectrum from the relatively benign isolated steatosis, defined as abnormal fat accumulation in greater than 5% of hepatocytes, to inflammation, then the progressive fibrosis, and eventually cirrhosis. Although there is no consensus on the exact cause, recent studies have contributed to a better understanding of this disease process.

Initial theories about the cause of MAFLD were based on the "two-hit" hypothesis. The "first-hit" was the accumulation of hepatic triglycerides in the setting of obesity and insulin resistance, which put the liver at risk for the "second-hit," which was inflammatory cytokines and oxidative stress that sets off a cascade leading to steatohepatitis and fibrosis.[9] This "two-hit" theory was later modified to include the possible role of free fatty acids. In patients with obesity and insulin resistance, there is an increased influx of free fatty acids into the liver. After undergoing β-oxidation or esterification with glycerol to form triglycerides within hepatocytes, free fatty acids are able to cause direct toxicity by increasing oxidative stress and activation of inflammatory cascades.[10]

However, even with the addition of the role free fatty acids play in the pathogenesis of MAFLD, the "two-hit" theory was too simplistic to explain the complex interaction between genetic and environmental factors that leads to the progression of MAFLD.

Thus, the "multiple-hit model" was developed. This model incorporates other factors, including genetic polymorphisms, epigenetics, bile acids, and microbiome.

Several polymorphisms have been implicated in the cause of MAFLD. Patatin-like phospholipase domain-containing protein 3 gene (PNPLA3) is a gene that encodes for adiponutrin, an enzyme present in liver and adipose tissue.[11] An isoleucine-to-methionine variant of PNPLAs (I148M) has been identified as a major determinant of liver fat content, as it increases lipogenic activity and impairs mobilization of triglycerides from hepatocyte lipid droplets.[12,13] Its role in development of MALFD in children and adolescents is currently being established with 1 study concluding that PNPLA3 I148M confers susceptibility to hepatic steatosis in obese youths without increasing the level of hepatic and peripheral insulin resistance.[14] Multiple studies suggest that PNPLA I148M may represent a general modifier of fibrogenesis in liver disease and, thus, it is important to identify the children with this polymorphism, as they are at a higher risk of progression to nonalcoholic steatohepatitis (NASH).[12]

A cytosine-to-thymine single-nucleotide polymorphism (SNP) in transmembrane 6 superfamily member 2 (TM6SF2) gives rise to the E167K variant. This variant decreases very-low-density lipoprotein–mediated lipid secretion and increases susceptibility to liver damage in children.[15] A cytosine-to-thymine SNP in the membrane-bound O-acyltransferase domain-containing protein 7 (MBOAT7) is associated with increased risk of fibrosis and, therefore, progression to NASH.

G protein–coupled receptor 120 (GPR120) is a receptor for polyunsaturated fatty acids (PUFAs) that is expressed mainly on adipocytes and Kupffer cells.[16] In adipose tissue, the interaction between GPR120 and PUFAs has an anti-inflammatory effect. A variant of GPR120, 270H, has been shown to reduce the signaling effects between GPR120 and PUFAs and thus decrease their anti-inflammatory effects.[17] One study, although underpowered, was able to show that adolescents carrying GPR120 270H had significantly higher ALT and ferritin levels than wild-type subjects.[16] Interestingly, this study also showed that subjects with coexisting GRP120 270H and PNPLA3 148M have significantly higher ALT levels than those with PNPLA3 148M alone. However, those subjects with wild-type PNPLA3 and GRP120 270H had normal ALT levels, thus further emphasizing the dynamic pathophysiology described in the "multiple-hit model."[16]

There are several other polymorphisms that have been found to be playing a role in the development of MAFLD and progression to NASH. These polymorphisms are involved in monosaccharide uptake, lipid synthesis, metabolism, lipid excretion, and insulin receptor activity.[13] However, the exact role of these polymorphisms and their degree of correlation with fibrogenesis is not well understood and requires more research, especially in the pediatric population.

PATHOPHYSIOLOGY

The development of steatosis begins with the accumulation of excess carbohydrate precursors. This stimulates the upregulation of de novo lipogenesis. A concurrent process is also occurring whereby increased fat intake from the diet is resulting in increased uptake of fatty acids from chylomicron particles, resulting in lipolysis. These processes together result in the accumulation of hepatic free fatty acids and triglycerides.[18]

These free fatty acids and triglycerides collect in the cytoplasm of hepatocytes and are supposed to be disposed of via mitochondrial β-oxidation. However, if this process becomes overwhelmed, it leads to the inadequate disposal of free fatty acids and increased production of toxic lipids, unesterified cholesterol, and ceramides that cause hepatotoxicity and increased inflammation.[18] Inflammation leads to the recruitment of multiple cytokines that contribute further to hepatocellular damage. The recruitment of Kupffer cells and activation of hepatic stellate cells result in fibrosis, cirrhosis, and possible hepatocellular carcinoma.[18]

Gut-liver axis is another important process that contributes to this complex system. Bile acids act as the regulators of this system by playing a key role in nutrient absorption and signal transduction to the liver via modulation of the gut microbiome and activation of various receptors. Bile acids act as crucial regulators of liver metabolism. The opposite is also true in that the liver is acting as a key regulator of intestinal homeostasis. Although the exact mechanisms are still an active area of research, an impaired gut-liver axis function has been implicated in the pathogenesis of MAFLD.[19]

This complex web of interconnected processes that leads to the development of MAFLD was discovered through research into adult MAFLD. However, the pathogenesis of pediatric MAFLD has not been given the same consideration. Thus, significant research is required to evaluate possible differences in the development of pediatric MAFLD.

PATHOLOGY AND CLASSIFICATION

Although the exact histologic criteria for adult NASH evolved over time, main features include the presence of macrovesicular steatosis, ballooning degeneration of hepatocytes, and a mix of lobular inflammation with or without a degree of portal inflammation.[20] There are some commonalities in the histopathology of adult and pediatric NASH; however, there are also some notable differences. A 2005 study of more than 100 pediatric patients with NALFD was first able to describe 2 distinct subsets of NASH in children.[21]

Type I NASH shows a similar histopathologic pattern to that of adult NASH. It is defined as the presence of steatosis with ballooning degeneration and/or perisinusoidal fibrosis in the absence of portal features.[21] **Fig. 3** highlights these characteristic features using hematoxylin-eosin (H&E) staining.

Type II or pediatric NASH is different from type I or adult NASH in that it is defined as the presence of steatosis along with portal inflammation and/or fibrosis in the absence of ballooning degeneration and perisinusoidal fibrosis, as shown in **Figs. 4** and **5**.[21] This type of NASH is more common overall but especially in male patients as well as in Asians, Native Americans and Hispanics.[20] The presence of portal inflammation, which is unique to type II NASH, has been independently associated with clinically significant fibrosis, suggesting this feature is predictive of a faster disease progression.[22]

Although there is a desire to make types I and II NASH distinct entities for simplicity's sake, there is also significant overlap. One case series demonstrated that 66% of patients with histologically diagnosed NASH fell into this overlapping category.[22] Although the exact percentage of each NASH type, as well as overlap, varies between studies and populations, more research is needed to clarify the natural history of each phenotype.

EVALUATION AND DIAGNOSIS

MAFLD should be suspected in any overweight or obese child with hepatic steatosis on imaging or liver biopsy with or without elevated ALT. However, it should not be assumed as the only cause. Certain conditions and medications may have similar presentation, and missing them may have serious consequences. MAFLD is currently considered a diagnosis of exclusion, and it can coexist with other conditions.[23]

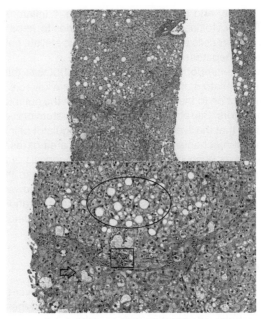

Fig. 3. Adult (type 1) NASH (H&E stain). Steatosis (*circle*), ballooned hepatocyte (*arrow*), inflammation (*square*). (*Courtesy of* Daniela Allende, MD, Cleveland, OH.)

Liver biopsy remains the gold standard to make the diagnosis of MAFLD. It also helps in assessing NASH activity and staging fibrosis. However, in reality, liver biopsy is not performed on every MAFLD patient, and its use is limited for certain indications, ruling out other causes for elevated liver enzymes, assessing NASH activity, and ruling out advanced fibrosis. Liver biopsy has its own limitations, including sampling bias, and the risk of complications, including hemorrhage and, rarely, death.[24]

Emerging noninvasive measures have become appealing in both adult and pediatric MAFLD. Those measures try to evaluate different aspects of the disease, including the presence of steatosis, steatosis grade, NASH activity, and of stage fibrosis. They are generally divided into biomarkers and imaging modalities. Several biomarkers have been developed in adult MAFLD, and few, like FIB-4, are recommended by adult

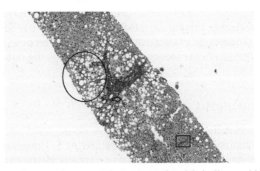

Fig. 4. Pediatric (type 2) NASH (H&E stain). Steatosis (*circle*), ballooned hepatocyte (*arrow*), inflammation (*square*). (*Courtesy of* Daniela Allende, MD, Cleveland, OH.)

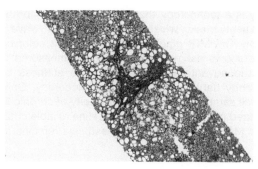

Fig. 5. Pediatric (type 2) NASH (Trichrome stain). (*Courtesy of* Daniela Allende, MD, Cleveland, OH.)

guidelines to screen patients at risk for significant fibrosis.[25,26] Unlike adult MAFLD, there is no reliable biomarker that made it to clinical practice in pediatric MAFLD. On the other hand, imaging modalities show promising results in both age groups.[27]

Conventional ultrasound (US) is a commonly used imaging modality that has been studied extensively. It is cheap, noninvasive, and well tolerated by children. Hepatic steatosis is generally suspected based on increased liver echogenicity compared with adjacent right renal parenchyma. It has shown very good accuracy to detect moderate to severe steatosis when compared with liver biopsy with area under the receiver operating characteristic curve of 0.87.[28] However, low sensitivity and specificity in detecting mild steatosis made it less favorable by the most recent North American Society for Pediatric Gastroenterology, Hepatology, and Nutrition recommendations as a tool to screen for the disease in at-risk children.[23] US is still recommended by the European guidelines as a screening tool.[29] New US-based modalities like quantitative US to detect and grade steatosis are being validated in adults.[30] Magnetic resonance proton density fat fraction (MR-PDFF) is a very accurate imaging tool to quantify liver fat. However, it is not very popular, is only available at tertiary centers, and is commonly used in clinical trials.

Velocity controlled transient elastography (VCTE) is emerging as a popular noninvasive modality to grade steatosis and stage fibrosis. It is a US-based technology that mechanically produces a low-frequency shear wave, which propagates through the liver. The velocity of the shear wave measured by the device correlates positively with liver stiffness, which is measured in kilopascal. The attenuation of that shear wave correlates positively with liver steatosis and is measured using CAP score (controlled attenuation parameter) in decibel per meter. CAP score cutoff for the presence of steatosis ranges between 225 and 241 dB/m based on 2 pediatric studies using biopsy and MR-PDFF as a reference, respectively.[31,32] Although steatosis grade does correlate with CAP score, however, specific cutoff to determine steatosis grade is more problematic owing to significant overlap between cutoff suggested by different studies.

Acoustic radiation force impulse (ARFI) is another US-based technology that is similar to VCTE in using a probe that creates a push pulse wave that propagates through the liver in velocity that correlates with liver stiffness. Stiffness is expressed in meters per second. ARFI differs from VCTE by the ability to choose a region of interest within which the stiffness is measured. This lowers the rate of unsuccessful readings compared with VCTE especially in obese patients and patients with ascites.[27]

MR elastography is a technology that uses MRI and a vibration source that is placed on the patient trunk, which creates a shear wave that propagates throughout the liver. The MRI machine then creates a color-coded map called an elastogram that shows estimated liver stiffness measured in kilopascal. MR elastography has the advantage of assessing the stiffness of the entire liver regardless of the body habitus with very good accuracy. Only a few pediatric studies exist.[33] Small sample size and heterogeneity of chronic liver diseases (besides MAFLD) included make it challenging to define reliable cutoff values to stage fibrosis in pediatric MAFLD. The need for anesthesia remains a limiting factor in young children.

MANAGEMENT AND LIMITATIONS

The goal of treatment of MAFLD is regression in steatosis, inflammation, and ultimately, fibrosis. The cornerstone of treatment of pediatric MAFLD is weight loss through dietary improvement and increased physical activity. The most recent guidelines published in 2017 from the North American Society of Pediatric Gastroenterology, Hepatology, and Nutrition recommends "lifestyle modifications to improve diet and increase physical activity as the first-line treatment for all children with NAFLD."[23] A weight reduction of as little as 1 kg has been shown to improve serum biomarkers of MAFLD in children; thus, many studies have been aimed at determining which diet works most effectively for weight reduction in children.[34]

Multiple studies have shown a decrease in adiposity among overweight and obese adolescents after reduction of sugar-sweetened beverages.[35,36] The addition of high-fructose corn syrup to these beverages acts as a stimulator of glycolysis, lipogenesis, and glucose production in the liver and thus contributes to the pathogenesis of MAFLD.[37] Research also indicates that the Mediterranean diet can reduce liver steatosis and improve insulin sensitivity even without weight loss; however, more research needs to be done in this area.[38] Ultimately, the most effective diet is the one that is able to be sustained over time.

Metformin and vitamin E have been studied extensively as possible treatments for pediatric MAFLD owing to their effect on insulin resistance and oxidative stress. The TONIC trial was a 2011 multicenter, phase 3, randomized, placebo-controlled trial that aimed to look at changes in ALT, changes in histologic features of MAFLD, and resolution of NASH after treatment with metformin or vitamin E. This well-powered study concluded that, although treatment with vitamin E showed some histologic improvements, neither metformin nor vitamin E was superior to placebo in attaining sustained reduction in ALT.[39]

Docosahexaenoic acid, fish oil, oral insulin sensitizers, ursodeoxycholic acid, probiotics, and carnitine have all also been studied as possible treatment options for pediatric MAFLD; however, none have been shown to add significantly to the treatment effect of lifestyle modifications alone.[13]

EVOLVING TREATMENTS

In the last several years, different classes of medications have been suggested and are currently being studied as possible treatments for MAFLD in adults. The role of these pharmacotherapies in the treatment of MAFLD in children and adolescents has yet to be determined. However, safety and efficacy have been demonstrated in adults, and studies in the pediatric population will follow soon.[15] **Table 1** outlines the current state of pharmacologic treatment of MAFLD in children and adolescents.

Table 1
Evolving treatment for pediatric metabolic-associated fatty liver disease

Drug	Category	Mechanism of Action/Target	Clinical Trial Phase	Limitations
Elafibranor	Alpha and delta peroxisome proliferator-activated receptor (PPAR) dual agonist (PPAR-α/δ)	• Insulin sensitizer • Improves lipid metabolism	Phase 2 in pediatrics	• Been shown to resolve NASH without worsening fibrosis in adult, but pediatric trials are still ongoing[40] • Adult phase 3 trial terminated due to lack of efficacy
Lanifibranor	Pan-PPAR agonist	• Insulin sensitizer (shown to be more efficacious than dual-PPAR agonists[41]) • Reduces liver fibrosis	Phase 3 in adults	• No pediatric trials
Resmetirom	Thyroid hormone receptor (THR) β-selective agonist	• Targets THR-β receptors in hepatocytes that impact serum cholesterol and triglyceride levels	Phase 3 in adults	• Current adult study shows improvement in ballooning and inflammation within hepatocytes without worsening fibrosis, but no studies in children
Selonsertib	Apoptosis signal-regulating kinase 1 (ASK1) inhibitor	• Inhibits the ASK1 pathway that results in inflammatory and profibrotic changes in the liver • ASK1 is upregulated in patients with NASH and correlates with degree of fibrosis[40]	Phase 3 in adults	• Randomized clinical trials have shown no antifibrotic effect in adult patients with bridging fibrosis or compensated cirrhosis due to NASH[42] • Adult phase 3 trial terminated due to lack of efficacy • No pediatric trials
Obeticholic acid	Farnesoid X receptor (FXR) agonist	• Agonizes the FXR receptor (a bile acid receptor that regulates hepatic and peripheral glucose metabolism), which results in balancing of de novo lipogenesis and fatty acid oxidation as well as anti-inflammatory effects[43]	Phase 3 in adults	• Results in improvement in fibrosis without worsening of NASH in adult patients with stage F2 or F3 fibrosis but there are no pediatric trials[44]

(continued on next page)

Table 1
(continued)

Drug	Category	Mechanism of Action/Target	Clinical Trial Phase	Limitations
Cenicriviroc	C-C chemokine receptor types 2 and 5 dual antagonist	• Inhibits a pathway that causes fibrogenesis by monocyte and macrophage recruitment to the inflamed tissue and activation on hepatic stellate cells[40] • Downstream target	Phase 3 in adults	• Adult phase 3 trial (AURORA) terminated due to lack of efficacy • No pediatric trials
Aramchol (3β-arachidyl amido cholanoic acid)	Partial inhibitor of hepatic stearoyl-CoA desaturase (SCD1)	• Fatty acid–bile acid conjugate that inhibits SCD1 and results in improved steatohepatitis, fibrosis, and steatosis[45]	Phase 3 in adults	• No pediatric trials
Semaglutide[a]	Glucagon-like peptide-1 analogue	• Increases postprandial insulin level in a glucose-dependent manner, reduces glucagon secretion, delays gastric emptying, and induces weight loss through appetite reduction and decreased energy intake[46]	Phase 3 in pediatrics	• No studies to date exploring direct effect on fatty liver disease (although a phase 3 pediatric study is actively recruiting MAFLD patients currently) • Requires weekly injection
Liraglutide	Glucagon-like peptide-1 analogue	• Increases postprandial insulin level in a glucose-dependent manner, reduces glucagon secretion, delays gastric emptying, and induces weight loss through appetite reduction and decreased energy intake[46]	Phase 3 in pediatrics	• No published studies to date exploring direct effect on fatty liver disease • Requires daily injections

[a] Oral version (Rybelsus) has been proven to have similar efficacy and tolerability in adults but no research is available in pediatrics.

SUMMARY

MAFLD in children and adolescents is a problem that is only growing in scale. Although there are promising therapies on the horizon, patient risk stratification continues to pose a challenge owing to limited data on the disease's natural history in this population. Tackling this growing pandemic in children will certainly have a positive impact on the future of adult MAFLD and its economic burden.

CLINICS CARE POINTS

- Increased awareness of metabolic-associated fatty liver disease in children and adolescents can lead to early diagnosis and intervention.
- There are several noninvasive modalities, such as ultrasound and elastography, that can help assist in grading steatosis and staging fibrosis.
- Lifestyle changes and weight loss remain the mainstay of treatment for pediatric metabolic-associated fatty liver disease.
- Emerging therapies that target varied steps in the pathogenesis of metabolic-associated fatty liver disease may play a larger role in treatment in the near future.

DISCLOSURES

The authors have nothing to disclose.

REFERENCES

1. Zhang X, Wu M, Liu Z, et al. Increasing prevalence of NAFLD/NASH among children, adolescents and young adults from 1990 to 2017: A population-based observational study. BMJ Open 2021;11(5):e042843.
2. Obesity and overweight. World Health Organization. Available at: https://www.who.int/news-room/fact-sheets/detail/obesity-and-overweight. Accessed January 28, 2023.
3. Obita G, Alkhatib A. Disparities in the Prevalence of Childhood Obesity-Related Comorbidities: A Systematic Review. Front Public Health 2022;10. https://doi.org/10.3389/fpubh.2022.923744.
4. Yi M, Peng W, Feng X, et al. Extrahepatic morbidities and mortality of NAFLD: an umbrella review of meta-analyses. Aliment Pharmacol Ther 2022 Oct;56(7):1119–30.
5. Anderson EL, Howe LD, Jones HE, et al. The prevalence of non-alcoholic fatty liver disease in children and adolescents: A systematic review and meta-analysis. PLoS One 2015;10(10).
6. Castillo-Leon E, Cioffi CE, Vos MB. Perspectives on youth-onset nonalcoholic fatty liver disease. Endocrinol Diabetes Metab 2020;3(4). https://doi.org/10.1002/edm2.184.
7. Younossi ZM, Koenig AB, Abdelatif D, et al. Global Epidemiology of Nonalcoholic Fatty Liver Disease-Meta-Analytic Assessment of Prevalence, Incidence, and Outcomes. Hepatology 2016 Jul;64(1):73–84.
8. Hirode G, Saab S, Wong RJ. Trends in the Burden of Chronic Liver Disease among Hospitalized US Adults. JAMA Netw Open 2020;3(4). https://doi.org/10.1001/jamanetworkopen.2020.1997.

9. Fang YL, Chen H, Wang CL, et al. Pathogenesis of non-alcoholic fatty liver disease in children and adolescence: From "two hit theory" to "multiple hit model. World J Gastroenterol 2018;24(27):2974–83.

10. Dowman JK, Tomlinson JW, Newsome PN. Pathogenesis of non-alcoholic fatty liver disease. QJM 2009;103(2):71–83.

11. Marzuillo P, Grandone A, Perrone L, et al. Understanding the pathophysiological mechanisms in the pediatric non-alcoholic fatty liver disease: The role of genetics. World J Hepatol 2015;7(11):1439–43.

12. Dongiovanni P, Donati B, Fares R, et al. PNPLA3 I148M polymorphism and progressive liver disease. World J Gastroenterol 2013;19(41):6969–78.

13. Draijer L, Benninga M, Koot B. Pediatric NAFLD: an overview and recent developments in diagnostics and treatment. Expert Rev Gastroenterol Hepatol 2019; 13(5):447–61.

14. Santoro N, Kursawe R, D'Adamo E, et al. A common variant in the patatin-like phospholipase 3 gene (PNPLA3) is associated with fatty liver disease in obese children and adolescents. Hepatology 2010;52(4):1281–90.

15. Nobili V, Alisi A, Valenti L, et al. NAFLD in children: new genes, new diagnostic modalities and new drugs. Nat Rev Gastroenterol Hepatol 2019;16(9):517–30.

16. Marzuillo P, Grandone A, Conte M, et al. Novel association between a nonsynonymous variant (R270H) of the G-protein-coupled receptor 120 and liver injury in children and adolescents with obesity. J Pediatr Gastroenterol Nutr 2014;59(4): 472–5.

17. Oh DY, Talukdar S, Bae EJ, et al. GPR120 Is an Omega-3 Fatty Acid Receptor Mediating Potent Anti-inflammatory and Insulin-Sensitizing Effects. Cell 2010; 142(5):687–98.

18. Phen C, Ramirez CM. Hepatic Steatosis in the Pediatric Population: An Overview of Pathophysiology, Genetics, and Diagnostic Workup. Clin Liver Dis 2021;17(3): 191–5.

19. Xue R, Su L, Lai S, et al. Bile acid receptors and the gut–liver axis in nonalcoholic fatty liver disease. Cells 2021;10(11). https://doi.org/10.3390/cells10112806.

20. Carter-Kent C, Yerian LM, Brunt EM, et al. Nonalcoholic steatohepatitis in children: A multicenter clinicopathological study. Hepatology 2009;50(4):1113–20.

21. Schwimmer JB, Behling C, Newbury R, et al. Histopathology of pediatric nonalcoholic fatty liver disease. Hepatology 2005;42(3):641–9.

22. Mann JP, Valenti L, Scorletti E, et al. Nonalcoholic Fatty Liver Disease in Children. Semin Liver Dis 2018;38(1):1–13.

23. Vos MB, Abrams SH, Barlow SE, et al. NASPGHAN Clinical Practice Guideline for the Diagnosis and Treatment of Nonalcoholic Fatty Liver Disease in Children: Recommendations from the Expert Committee on NAFLD (ECON) and the North American Society of Pediatric Gastroenterology, Hepatology and Nutrition (NASPGHAN). J Pediatr Gastroenterol Nutr 2017;64(2):319–34.

24. Ovchinsky N, Moreira RK, Lefkowitch JH, et al. Liver Biopsy in Modern Clinical Practice: A Pediatric Point-of-View. 2012. Available at: http://www.anatomic.

25. Cusi K, Isaacs S, Barb D, et al. American Association of Clinical Endocrinology Clinical Practice Guideline for the Diagnosis and Management of Nonalcoholic Fatty Liver Disease in Primary Care and Endocrinology Clinical Settings: Co-Sponsored by the American Association for the Study of Liver Diseases (AASLD). Endocr Pract 2022;28(5):528–62.

26. Castera L, Friedrich-Rust M, Loomba R. Noninvasive Assessment of Liver Disease in Patients With Nonalcoholic Fatty Liver Disease. Gastroenterology 2019; 156(5):1264–81.e4.

27. Chen BR, Pan CQ. Non-invasive assessment of fibrosis and steatosis in pediatric non-alcoholic fatty liver disease. Clin Res Hepatol Gastroenterol 2022;46(1). https://doi.org/10.1016/j.clinre.2021.101755.

28. Shannon A, Alkhouri N, Carter-Kent C, et al. Ultrasonographic quantitative estimation of hepatic steatosis in children With NAFLD. J Pediatr Gastroenterol Nutr 2011;53(2):190–5.

29. Vajro P, Lenta S, Socha P, et al. Diagnosis of nonalcoholic fatty liver disease in children and adolescents: Position paper of the ESPGHAN hepatology committee. J Pediatr Gastroenterol Nutr 2012;54(5):700–13.

30. Lin SC, Heba E, Wolfson T, et al. Noninvasive diagnosis of nonalcoholic fatty liver disease and quantification of liver fat using a new quantitative ultrasound technique. Clin Gastroenterol Hepatol 2015;13(7):1337–45.e6.

31. Shin NY, Kim MJ, Lee MJ, et al. Transient elastography and sonography for prediction of liver fibrosis in infants with biliary atresia. J Ultrasound Med 2014;33(5): 853–64.

32. Desai NK, Harney S, Raza R, et al. Comparison of controlled attenuation parameter and liver biopsy to assess hepatic steatosis in pediatric patients. J Pediatr 2016;173:160–4.e1.

33. Xanthakos SA, Podb: resky DJ, Serai SD, et al. Use of magnetic resonance elastography to assess hepatic fibrosis in children with chronic liver disease. J Pediatr 2014;164(1):186–8.

34. Friesen CS, Hosey-Cojocari C, Chan SS, et al. Efficacy of Weight Reduction on Pediatric Nonalcoholic Fatty Liver Disease: Opportunities to Improve Treatment Outcomes Through Pharmacotherapy. Front Endocrinol 2021;12. https://doi.org/ 10.3389/fendo.2021.663351.

35. Ebbeling CB, Feldman HA, Chomitz VR, et al. A Randomized Trial of Sugar-Sweetened Beverages and Adolescent Body Weight. N Engl J Med 2012; 367(15):1407–16.

36. de Ruyter JC, Olthof MR, Seidell JC, et al. A Trial of Sugar-free or Sugar-Sweetened Beverages and Body Weight in Children. N Engl J Med 2012; 367(15):1397–406.

37. Taskinen MR, Packard CJ, Borén J. Dietary fructose and the metabolic syndrome. Nutrients 2019;11(9). https://doi.org/10.3390/nu11091987.

38. Ryan MC, Itsiopoulos C, Thodis T, et al. The Mediterranean Diet Improves Hepatic Steatosis and Insulin Sensitivity in Individuals with Non-Alcoholic Fatty Liver Disease. J Hepatol 2013;59(1):138–43.

39. Lavine JE, Schwimmer JB, van Natta ML, et al. Effect of Vitamin E or Metformin for Treatment of Nonalcoholic Fatty Liver Disease in Children and Adolescents The TONIC Randomized Controlled Trial. JAMA 2011;305(16):1659–68. Available at: https://jamanetwork.com/.

40. Crudele A, Panera N, Braghini MR, et al. The pharmacological treatment of nonalcoholic fatty liver disease in children. Expert Rev Clin Pharmacol 2020;13(11): 1219–27.

41. Francque SM, Bedossa P, Ratziu V, et al. A Randomized, Controlled Trial of the Pan-PPAR Agonist Lanifibranor in NASH. N Engl J Med 2021;385(17):1547–58.

42. Harrison SA, Wong VWS, Okanoue T, et al. Selonsertib for patients with bridging fibrosis or compensated cirrhosis due to NASH: Results from randomized phase III STELLAR trials. J Hepatol 2020;73(1):26–39.

43. Attia SL, Softic S, Mouzaki M. Evolving Role for Pharmacotherapy in NAFLD/ NASH. Clin Transl Sci 2021;14(1):11–9.

44. Younossi ZM, Ratziu V, Loomba R, et al. Obeticholic acid for the treatment of non-alcoholic steatohepatitis: interim analysis from a multicentre, randomised, placebo-controlled phase 3 trial. Lancet 2019;394(10215):2184–96.
45. Ratziu V, de Guevara L, Safadi R, et al. Aramchol in patients with nonalcoholic steatohepatitis: a randomized, double-blind, placebo-controlled phase 2b trial. Nat Med 2021;27(10):1825–35.
46. Kelly AS, Auerbach P, Barrientos-Perez M, et al. A randomized, controlled trial of liraglutide for adolescents with obesity. N Engl J Med 2020;382(22): 2117–28.

Lean Metabolic-Associated Fatty Liver Disease

Cameron Gofton, BSCi, MBBS, MPH, FRACP[a,b], McCawley Clark-Dickson, BMed, FRACP[b],
Jacob George, MBBS, PhD, FRACP[c,d,*]

KEYWORDS

- MAFLD • Lean MAFLD • Hepatic and extrahepatic MAFLD complications
- Lean MAFLD mortality

KEY POINTS

- Lean metabolic-associated fatty liver disease (MAFLD) is a distinct clinical entity that carries similar complication rates to overweight/obese MAFLD.
- Most studies addressing lean MAFLD have been performed as a subgroup analysis of larger data sets.
- More work needs to be performed in lean MAFLD to better understand the pathophysiology and response to management strategies.

INTRODUCTION

Fatty liver infiltration has been recognized for centuries. Early work by Ludwig and colleagues[1] resulted in a report examining the histologic similarities between alcohol-related liver disease and liver disease in the absence of a history of alcohol use, and thus the term nonalcoholic fatty liver disease (NAFLD) was born. Since that time, significant work has been undertaken to determine the pathophysiologic manifestations and clinical associations of this disorder, which differ from that of alcohol-related liver disease. However, the term NAFLD has persisted despite its inadequacies in describing the disease and its diagnostic characteristics.[2]

A nomenclature change for fatty liver disease was proposed in 2020 to replace NAFLD with a term that better reflects the known pathophysiology.[3] The international consensus used a 2-stage Delphi method and suggested the name metabolic (dysfunction) -associated fatty liver disease (MAFLD) and subsequently proposed a

[a] Royal North Shore Hospital, Level 4, Acute Services Building, St Leonards, Sydney, NSW 2065, Australia; [b] Gastroenterology and Hepatology, Bankstown-Lidcombe Hospital, Eldridge Road, Bankstown, NSW 2200, Australia; [c] University of Sydney, Sydney, Australia; [d] Gastroenterology and Hepatology, Westmead Hospital, Westmead, Australia
* Corresponding author. Storr Liver Centre, Westmead Institute for Medical Research, Westmead Hospital, Hawksbury Road, Westmead, NSW 2145.
E-mail address: Jacob.George@sydney.edu.au

Endocrinol Metab Clin N Am 52 (2023) 431–444
https://doi.org/10.1016/j.ecl.2023.02.003   endo.theclinics.com

simple set of criteria for diagnosis. Since the proposed change, there have been more than 1000 original articles referencing the name, inspiring a new wave of study into this field.

An aspect of MAFLD that has developed significantly since the introduction of the new classification has been studies on the clinical phenotype of lean MAFLD.[4] Reports before the introduction of MAFLD have shown that lean NAFLD is phenotypically different from overweight/obese NAFLD. Interestingly, individuals with normal weight with hepatic steatosis under the definition of NAFLD had similar outcomes as individuals who were overweight or obese, which may have been confounded by selection bias, underestimation of alcohol intake, and unaccounted weight changes over time.[6] Since the introduction of MAFLD into the diagnostic terminology, there have been several studies that have examined the associated pathophysiologic features and end-organ complications that accompany lean MAFLD.

DEFINITION OF LEAN METABOLIC-ASSOCIATED FATTY LIVER DISEASE

With the introduction of MAFLD into the medical nomenclature in 2020, simple diagnostic criteria were proposed.[3] Using the requisite hepatic steatosis of $\geq 5\%$ that makes up an NAFLD diagnosis, 3 nonexclusive diagnostic phenotypes were reported. The first MAFLD phenotype consisted of patients with an underlying diagnosis of type 2 diabetes who may or may not be of healthy body weight by body mass index (BMI) criteria. The second phenotype uses definitions of overweight/obesity by ethnic-specific BMI classifications, namely a BMI of 25 to 29.9 kg/m^2 for overweight and BMI of ≥ 30 kg/m^2 for obese individuals of European ancestry and a BMI of 23.0 to 24.9 kg/m^2 for overweight and BMI of ≥ 25 kg/m^2 for obesity in individuals of Asian descent. The third MAFLD phenotype consists of patients who are of healthy weight by ethnic-specific BMI criteria but who have metabolic dysregulatory factors that are part of the operational definition of metabolic syndrome. For a diagnosis of MAFLD using this criterion, an individual needs 2 of 7 risk factors. The risk factors include waist circumference, blood pressure, plasma triglycerides, plasma HDL-cholesterol, prediabetes, homeostasis model assessment of insulin resistance score, and plasma high-sensitivity C-reactive protein. Individuals require 1 of the 3 different phenotypes coupled with hepatic steatosis of $\geq 5\%$ for a diagnosis of MAFLD.[3] A unique aspect of the MAFLD criteria is that it provides an operational definition of what the disease is, rather than what it is not. Stemming from this, MAFLD can coexist with any other liver disease and contribute to its clinical manifestations and natural history. **Fig. 1** shows the graphical representation of MAFLD definition.

Although a definition of lean MAFLD was proposed in the initial diagnostic criteria as normal/lean weight with at least 2 metabolic dysregulatory risk factors, its utilization seemingly excludes patients of normal weight with diabetes and MAFLD.[3] The definition of lean MAFLD in this article uses either the first (if a patient is of health body weight with type 2 diabetes) or the third metabolic dysregulatory phenotype but not the second. Although commonly referred to as lean MAFLD, a more appropriate term would be that of MAFLD in lean/healthy-weight individuals.

PREVALENCE

Because of the short period of time between the introduction of MAFLD into the medical compendium and this publication, there have been limited data on the global prevalence of lean MAFLD.[4] Because of the high concordance between the diagnosis of NAFLD and MAFLD, previous studies have used this information to estimate the global

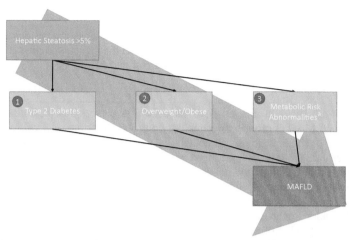

Fig. 1. Diagnostic criterion for MAFLD.[a]Metabolic risk abnormalities – 2 out of 7: Waist circumference >102/88 in Caucasian men and women, (or >90/80cm in Asian men or women). Blood pressure >130/85mmHg or specific drug treatment. Plasma triglycerides >150mg/dL (>1.70mmol/L) or specific drug treatment. Plasma HDL-cholesterol <40mg/dl (<1.0mmol/L) for men and <50mg/dl (<1.3mmol/L) for women or specific drug treatment. Prediabetes (i.e. fasting glucose levels 100-125mg/dL (5.6-6.9mmol/L) or 2-hour post-load glucose levels 140-199mg/dL (7.8-11.0mmol/L) of HbA1c of 5.7-6.4% (39-47mmol/mol). Homeostasis model assessment of insulin resistance score >2.5. Plasma high-sensitivity C-reactive protein level >2mg/L.

prevalence of MAFLD. In a study by Ye and colleagues,[5] a meta-analysis was conducted using 10,530,308 patients from 84 studies to estimate the global prevalence of lean NAFLD. In that study, lean NAFLD prevalence in the general population was 5.1%, with a prevalence of 19.2% in the global NAFLD population.

In another study by Chan and colleagues,[7] a meta-analysis and systematic review of 3,320,108 individuals were performed. Although it attempted to tabulate the global prevalence of MAFLD, owing to a lack of available data, there was limited insight into the prevalence of lean MAFLD. In a pooled analysis of 7106 patients from the 3,320,108 patients that the study reviewed, the prevalence of lean MAFLD was 5.4% of the general population. Although this is similar in numbers to previous studies, this estimate may be flawed particularly because of the geographic disparity of lean MAFLD demonstrated in the lean studies.

Several reports have attempted to examine the prevalence of MAFLD in order to identify the prevalence of lean MAFLD.[4,6–15] These studies have led to a wide range of lean MAFLD prevalence estimates ranging from 3.1% to 7.9% in the general population, and between 3.0% and 35.0% for prevalence within the wider MAFLD population. There are significant ethnic disparities in the reported prevalence and incidence owing to the wider uptake of MAFLD terminology among Asian countries, with less reported data from the West.[4,6–15] At this time, the prevalence and incidence of lean MAFLD appear to be similar to that of lean NAFLD; however, significantly more data in this area are required to establish a better global and ethnic estimation of the burden of this disease. It should also be noted that most studies have not determined the prevalence of lean MAFLD in patients with a coexistent secondary liver disease, which may be significantly underestimated in areas of high prevalence of chronic liver disease, such as alcohol-related liver disease.

PATHOPHYSIOLOGIC CHARACTERISTICS

Although little is known about lean MAFLD clinicopathologic characteristics, there have been several recent studies that have examined the clinical features of the condition and its metabolic and nonmetabolic associations (**Table 1**).

Disease Associations

For lean MAFLD, several articles have assessed its clinicopathologic associations compared with MAFLD groups and healthy controls. Unfortunately, because of the heterogeneity of these studies, particularly in view of the ethnic disparities in lean MAFLD, there are limited data, and that data appear at times to be conflicting.

In a recent study by Chan and colleagues[7] from the pooled analysis of 7100 patients with a prevalence of lean MAFLD of 5.4%, the associated clinicopathologic features were determined. Compared with healthy controls, patients with lean MAFLD were significantly older (mean difference [MD], 2.22; $P = .0001$), were more frequent in men (odds ratio [OR], 1.68; $P = .0003$), and were related to metabolic complications, such as hypertension (OR, 2.63; $P<.0001$) and type 2 diabetes (OR, 3.80; $P<.0001$). Although the correlation between type 2 diabetes and hypertension coincides with the determination of lean MAFLD as per the diagnostic criterion, the higher prevalence in older and male patients appears to be significant when compared with healthy controls in the largest study addressing this issue to date.

Cheng and colleagues[16] investigated 394 patients diagnosed with MAFLD, of which 65 (16.5%) were defined as lean MAFLD. This study compared individuals with lean MAFLD with healthy controls, and individuals with lean MAFLD with nonlean MAFLD. Factors that were independently associated with MAFLD in lean subjects were BMI (OR, 1.5; $P = .011$), waist circumference (OR, 1.1; $P = .010$), and hypertension (OR, 3.7; $P = .032$). Comparison between lean and nonlean MAFLD showed that the lean phenotype was associated with older age (61.1 years vs 57.5 years), female sex (69.2% vs 42.9%), higher high-density lipoprotein (47.8 mg/dL vs 42.0 mg/dL; $P<.001$), but lower waist circumference (76.8 cm vs 90.34 cm $\pm$ 8.75 cm; $P<.001$), diastolic blood pressure (75.5 mm Hg vs 79.47 mm Hg; $P = .008$), serum triglycerides (116.8 mg/dL vs 143.33 mg/dL; $P = .015$), and alanine aminotransferase levels (33.8 U/L vs 42.38 U/L; $P = .001$). Variables that were significant on binary logistic regression were age (1.4; $P = .040$) and waist circumference (OR, 0.81 95%; $P<.001$).[7]

Several extrahepatic complications have been associated in the wider MAFLD population, including chronic kidney disease, breast cancer, colorectal cancer, polycystic ovarian syndrome, and cardiac arrhythmias; these data are not readily available for the lean MAFLD subgroup.[17–19] Further research thus needs to be performed to assess for disease associations that are associated with lean MAFLD. At this stage, the literature on lean MAFLD is in its infancy, and further prospective evidence will further elaborate on clinicopathologic features.

Liver Fibrosis

Individuals with lean MAFLD have conflicting evidence when it comes to levels of fibrosis and noninvasive liver fibrosis scores. The main scoring systems that have been used in the NAFLD literature are the NAFLD fibrosis score (NFS) and the Fibrosis-index 4 (FIB-4). These systems have been extensively validated in NAFLD populations, and recent evidence in the wider MAFLD population suggests that these scores work as well to exclude significant fibrosis.[20]

Younes and colleagues[21] examined 1339 biopsy-proven MAFLD subjects of white ethnicity from 4 countries and showed that the prevalence of lean MAFLD was

Table 1
Clinicopathologic features of lean metabolic–associated fatty liver disease

Study		Patients	Results
Lin et al,[28] 2021	Total MAFLD	341	Compared with all MAFLD, lean MAFLD were:
	Lean MAFLD	28	• Older age, 60.7 ± 9.2 y vs 55.8 ± 10.2 y (P = .015)
			• Higher prevalence of diabetes 67.9% vs 28.8% (P<.001)
			• Lower serum ALT 33.2 ± 15.7 vs 48.1 ± 38.9 (P = .048)
			• Lower BMI 21.4 ± 1.4 vs 27.1 ± 3.0 (P<.001)
Zeng et al,[15] 2022	Total MAFLD	3340	Compared with all MAFLD, lean diabetic MAFLD had a higher prevalence of
	Lean MAFLD	1171	advanced fibrosis (14.7%)
Yu et al,[13] 2022	Lean MAFLD	531	Compared with lean NAFLD, lean MAFLD were:
	Lean NAFLD	816	• Older age, higher weight circumference, and high prevalence of diabetes
			(P<.001)
			• Higher AST (35.39 ± 18.97 vs 32.19 ± 11.41; P = .0034)
			• High FPG (5.84 ± 1.77 vs 5.50 ± 1.48; P = .030)
Yuan et al,[14] 2022	Total MAFLD	49,734	Compared with all MAFLD, lean MAFLD had a higher female predominance
	Lean MAFLD	724	(62.43% vs 47.30%; P<.001)
Ordonez-Vazquez et al,[6] 2022	Lean MAFLD	118	Compared with lean NAFLD, lean MAFLD had:
	Lean NAFLD	273	• Older age (OR, 1.42; 95% CI, 1.02–1.97; P = .036)
			• Higher fasting glucose (OR, 1.80; 95% CI, 1.30–2.48; P<.0001)
			• Higher triglycerides (OR, 1.52; 95% CI, 1.12–2.08; P = .007)
			• Higher waist circumference (OR, 2.04; 95% CI, 1.47–2.83; P<.0001)
Chan et al,[7] 2022	Total patients	7100	Compared with general population, lean MAFLD had:
	Lean MAFLD	381	• Older age (MD, 2.22; 95% CI, 1.09–3.336; P = .0001)
			• Male predominance (OR, 1.68; 95% CI, 1.27–2.21; P = .0003)
			• Higher prevalence of diabetes (OR, 3.80; 95% CI, 1.74–2.38; P<.001)

(continued on next page)

Table 1
(continued)

Study	Patients		Results
Cheng et al,[16] 2021	Total MAFLD	329	Compared with all MAFLD, lean MAFLD had:
	Lean MAFLD	65	• Older age (61.1 ± 8.01 y vs 57.5 ± 10.57 y; *P* = .001)
			• Female predominance (69.2% vs 42.9%; *P*<.001)
			• Higher HDL (47.81 mg/dL ± 11.45 mg/dL vs 42.02 mg/dL ± 11.83 mg/dL; *P*<.001)
			• Lower waist circumference (76.86 cm ± 5.27 cm vs 90.34 cm ± 8.75 cm; *P*<.001)
			• Lower diastolic blood pressure (75.51 mm Hg ± 9.80 mm Hg vs 79.47 mm Hg ± 11.13 mm Hg; *P* = .008)
			• Lower serum triglycerides (116.80 mg/dL ± 66.14 mg/dL vs 143.33 mg/dL ± 82.65 mg/dL; *P* = .015)
			• Lower ALT (33.77U/L ± 16.50 U/L vs 42.38U/L ± 27.36U/L; *P* = .001)

14.4% out of the total population of MAFLD. When reviewed in detail, patients with lean MAFLD had less severe disease with lower prevalence of metabolic syndrome (54.1% vs 71.2%; $P<.001$), lower proportions with advanced fibrosis (10.1% vs 25.2%; $P<.001$), and a lower prevalence of type 2 diabetes (9.2% vs 31.4%; $P<.001$).

In a more recent study by Eren and colleagues,[22] the accuracy of FIB-4 and NFS was assessed against liver biopsies in patients with MAFLD stratified by BMI. In lean MAFLD, the area under the receiver operating curve failed to discriminate patients with advanced fibrosis using FIB-4 ($P = .352$) and NFS ($P = .511$), and they suggested that new noninvasive markers for advanced fibrosis were needed for lean MAFLD. Unfortunately, there are issues with this blanket statement that are not addressed in the article. There were only 4 patients with lean MAFLD who had advanced fibrosis on biopsy out of a total of 37 patients. Although this study is otherwise reasonable, it is clearly not powered to provide reliable data to answer the question.

From established evidence regarding noninvasive fibrosis markers in lean NAFLD patients and the overlap of lean NAFLD and lean MAFLD, it would appear that FIB-4 and NFS should have reasonable ability to exclude advanced fibrosis in the latter population.[23,24] The conflicting evidence regarding noninvasive biomarkers' ability to discriminate advanced fibrosis from nonadvanced fibrosis in the lean MAFLD population has not been adequately addressed in the literature at this time.

Genetics

The contribution of genetic variation to pathogenic liver fat infiltration has been an area of keen research interest. Although genetic variants have an impact on fatty liver disease, the exact pathophysiologic mechanisms underpinning the higher prevalence of liver fat in these patients have not been fully elucidated. The change in nomenclature has been a driver to reexamine the genetic variants and their association with MAFLD. Further to this, the subgroup of lean MAFLD has been examined to determine the weight that these known genetic variants have on the underlying disease process, and on hepatic and extrahepatic complications.

In the study performed by Younes and colleagues,[21] genetic analysis was performed on the genetic variant PNPLA3 I1448M. The study showed no differences in the PNPLA3 I1148M ($P = .57$) between patients with lean MAFLD and patients with nonlean MAFLD.[21] Similarly, another study by Liu and colleagues[25] examined for outcomes of MAFLD in terms of liver cancer, cirrhosis, other liver disease, cardiovascular disease, renal diseases, and other cancers from the UK BioBank coupled with the genetic variants previously reported for NAFLD. A subgroup analysis was performed on patients with lean MAFLD and showed that they had higher rates of hepatocellular carcinoma (hazard ratio [HR], 3.23), cirrhosis (HR, 11.73), other liver disease (HR, 4.46), cardiovascular disease (HR, 1.37), renal disease (HR, 1.53), and other cancers (HR, 1.18).

Interestingly, the genetic variants had an increased impact in MAFLD on the above-mentioned complications but did not have an associated effect on patients with lean MAFLD.[25] Although this suggests some interesting pathophysiologic nuances surrounding the lean MAFLD phenotype, there were several issues that limit its applicability to practice. First, because of lack of imaging data, hepatic steatosis was implied by noninvasive biomarkers using the fatty liver index. Although this has been used in previous studies and shown to have relatively good sensitivity, it is not part of the usual diagnostic pathway for MAFLD. Second, the aforementioned complications were assessed on the basis of patients' ICD codes, rather than review of the patients or formal interrogation of the medical notes.

Although genetic variations do appear to have a place in the wider MAFLD population, currently their impact on lean MAFLD appears to be conflicting. The investigators of the previous studies have suggested that genetic variations appear to play a greater role in peripheral fat accumulation and that may influence their impact on both the hepatic and the extrahepatic complications of lean MAFLD. From previous studies examining NAFLD, there is a suggestion that genetic factors may have an effect; however, this is less pronounced in the absence of environmental factors, such as a sedentary lifestyle or poor diet.[26] At this time, there is a lack of evidence on genetic factors and their impact on lean MAFLD, and further research is required.

Dual Causes

One of the most significant features of the MAFLD definition is the removal of exclusion of coexisting liver diseases that was a prerequisite for an NAFLD diagnosis. This has allowed individuals to assess comorbid MAFLD with other liver diseases, such as viral hepatitis and autoimmune disease, and the relevant associations and complications of dual cause liver disease.

Al-Omary and colleagues[27] studied patients admitted to 2 tertiary institutions who underwent a liver biopsy for MAFLD and chronic hepatitis C. In the review period, there were 437 patients with MAFLD and 321 patients with dual MAFLD and chronic hepatitis C.[27] This study demonstrated that dual MAFLD and chronic hepatitis C had higher rates of advanced fibrosis over those with chronic hepatitis C alone (32.7% vs 14.2%; $P<.001$), A subgroup analysis of those with chronic hepatitis C was performed comparing patients with lean MAFLD with overweight/obese MAFLD and diabetic MAFLD, with comparable rates of advanced fibrosis (30.0% vs 31.9% vs 42.9%; $P = .352$).[27] This demonstrates that the overall rates of advanced fibrosis are higher with dual causes when combined with MAFLD and affect those with lean as well as overweight/obese individuals.

A recent study by Lin and colleagues[28] reviewed patients with chronic hepatitis B with Barcelona Clinic Liver Cancer (BCLC) 0/A hepatocellular carcinoma undergoing hepatic resection for presence of MAFLD. Of the 812 patients who underwent hepatic resection, 369 had MAFLD, with 28 satisfying the criteria for lean MAFLD. In multivariate analysis, lean MAFLD was associated with a higher risk of hepatocellular carcinoma recurrence when compared with nonlean MAFLD (HR, 2.03; $P = .020$) independent of other predictive risk factors.

Although these findings are useful and highlight the contributory effect of lean MAFLD on viral hepatitis, further work is required to establish disease synergisms in healthy-weight individuals.

Associated Complications and Prognosis

As with the aforementioned areas in lean MAFLD, the level of evidence surrounding prognosis is scarce and misleading. Because of the relatively novel nature of the nomenclature, currently all the data are retrospective from previously collected databases. Because of this, there are critical data flaws in most of the studies presented, which hamper their direct applicability to patient care.

Several complications have been highlighted as associations with lean MAFLD in recent reports. In a study by Fukunaga and colleagues,[29] 9100 patients who underwent esophagogastroduodendoscopy and ultrasonography were reviewed and placed into MAFLD and non-MAFLD groups. MAFLD was diagnosed in 26.5% of patients in the study. Interestingly, stratification analysis showed that the cumulative incidence of reflux esophagitis was significantly higher in lean MAFLD when compared with the nonlean MAFLD group (HR, 1.33). On logistic regression, visceral adiposity was the only independent metabolic risk factor for reflux esophagitis (HR, 2.83; P = .0457) in the lean MAFLD group.

In another study by Bessho and colleagues,[30] 977 patients with a previous diagnosis of NAFLD were evaluated for subclinical atherosclerosis using cardiac computed tomographic scans, brachial-ankle pulse-wave velocity, and carotid artery ultrasound as part of health checkup. Using these previously collected data, patients were reclassified into MAFLD criteria as overweight/obese, type 2 diabetic, or lean MAFLD. Overall, there were high rates of subclinical atherosclerosis across these groups. In particular, it showed that lean MAFLD had a positive coronary artery calcification score of greater than 0 (OR, 2.26; P = .006) and greater than 100 (OR, 3.48; P<.001), and carotid intimal thickness $\geq$1.1 (OR, 3.77; P<.001), all of which had higher OR than individuals who were diagnosed with overweight/obese MAFLD. Of particular note, those with lean MAFLD did not have increased brachial ankle pulse wave velocity greater than 1400, whereas those with diabetic MAFLD and overweight/obese MAFLD did.

A recent study be Peng and colleagues[31] examined the effects of MAFLD subgroups on left ventricular diastolic function and cardiac morphology. Of the 171 patients with MAFLD, 31 had lean MAFLD. Although both diabetic MAFLD and overweight/obese MAFLD had evidence of left ventricular diastolic dysfunction and cardiac remodeling, lean patients did not demonstrate any association. This is interesting, as there appears to be a different cardiovascular pathophysiologic pathway that the lean MAFLD phenotype exhibits when compared with diabetic and overweight/obese patients with MAFLD, although confirmation in other larger cohorts is warranted.

In a study by Lee and colleagues,[12] 8,412,730 participants in a nationwide health screening database were categorized into overweight/obese MAFLD, diabetic MAFLD, and lean MAFLD. The health screening substituted the fatty liver index for imaging demonstration of hepatic steatosis. Using this health screening at baseline, patients were followed up for a median of 10 years, and data were examined for incident cardiovascular disease risk, development of liver cancer, liver transplantation, and all-cause mortality. Of the total number of participants, 3,087,640 (36.7%) were given a diagnosis of MAFLD, with 2,424,086 (78.5%) classified as overweight MAFLD, 490,793 (16.0%) classified as diabetic MAFLD, and 170,761 (5.5%) classified as lean MAFLD.

Using overweight MAFLD as the control, lean MAFLD had the second highest increased risk when compared with diabetic MAFLD in cardiovascular disease events (HR, 1.41 vs HR, 2.16), liver cancer (HR, 1.52 vs HR, 2.42) and liver transplantation (HR, 1.93 vs HR, 1.98), but higher all-cause mortality (HR, 2.40 vs HR, 2.32). In addition, cardiovascular disease events increased significantly in lean MAFLD in the presence of advanced liver fibrosis compared with no advanced liver fibrosis (HR, 1.15 vs HR, 1.04). The investigators suggested that these results indicate that the fibrotic burden is a driver of cardiovascular disease risk, and this burden may be the driver for differences in liver-related outcomes.[12] Unfortunately, it is unclear from the data if there is an increased burden of other comorbidities affecting patients with lean MAFLD, which lead to their overall higher all-cause mortality, or whether lean MAFLD is the driver.

Further to the study by Younes and colleagues[21] mentioned above, the 1339 biopsy-proven patients with MAFLD were followed up for a median of 7.8 years. Although these individuals appeared to have less severe disease at baseline, their prognosis appears to be similar. There was no statistically significant difference between lean MAFLD and nonlean MAFLD in terms of liver-related events (4.7% vs 7.7%; $P = .37$) and survival ($P = .069$), although survival did trend toward significance. Despite this more favorable baseline metabolic profile in lean MAFLD, these patients experience both hepatic and extrahepatic complications of the disease, including hepatocellular carcinoma and cardiovascular disease.

In a study by Chen and colleagues,[32] patients from the NHANES III database were analyzed for mortality based on the specific MAFLD phenotype. This showed that lean MAFLD had increased mortality when compared with healthy subjects (HR, 1.4 95%; $P<.001$), which continued to be statistically significant when adjusted for major confounders. Although this study defined lean MAFLD as individuals without diabetes and who were not overweight or obese, and adjusted for metabolic conditions associated with the diagnosis of MAFLD, the increased mortality risk continued to be significant.

A study by Dao and colleagues[8] using the widely cited NHANES III, which has arguably the best long-term data for fatty liver disease, combined lean and overweight patients into a nonobese MAFLD category versus obese MAFLD. Patients with lean MAFLD made up 15% of the nonobese MAFLD category, with an overall prevalence of 7.2% in the total MAFLD population. The investigators showed that nonobese patients with MAFLD had a higher 20-year cumulative incidence for all-cause mortality compared with obese MAFLD (33.2% vs 28.8%; $P = .0137$). In this study, FIB-4 1.3 to 2.67, FIB-4 >2.67, and cardiovascular disease were the strongest risk factors associated with increased mortality (HR, 2.73; $P<.001$; HR, 3.69; $P<.001$; HR, 3.19; $P<.001$, respectively). Although the combination of lean and overweight into a nonobese category limits the applicability of the results in terms of the lean MAFLD population and must be interpreted with caution, there appears to be higher incidence rates of mortality in this phenotype.

Semmler and colleagues[33] reported on patients undergoing colorectal cancer screening. Of the 4718 patients, 221 (4.7%) fulfilled criteria for lean MAFLD. During a median follow-up of 7.5 years, 8.6% of patients with lean MAFLD died compared with 2.7% of patients with lean NAFLD and 5.6% of healthy controls. The main drivers of increased death in these patients were attributed to age and components of the metabolic syndrome. Unfortunately, there were some limitations in this study that decreased its utility in prescribing it to the lean MAFLD population. First, as part of the trial design, other coexisting liver diseases and alcohol consumption were excluded. Unlike NAFLD, MAFLD needs not exclude concomitant liver diseases, which limits the utilization of this study to the real-world lean MAFLD population. The second is that components of the metabolic syndrome cannot be used in an adjustment model for MAFLD, as they are used to formulate the MAFLD diagnosis. Removing these components invalidates the diagnosis of MAFLD, and the resultant assessment using adjustment modeling was assessing steatosis (**Fig. 2**).

TREATMENTS

The mainstay of treatment of lean MAFLD at this time is the same as for nonlean MAFLD. Lifestyle modifications centering on diet and exercise form the bedrock of management for this chronic disease. Although this has been proven to be effective among the lean NAFLD population to decrease hepatic steatosis, there has yet to be a study performed that addresses the lean MAFLD population to examine the effectiveness of these interventions, as also the long-term outcomes.

Currently there are no approved drug therapies available for MAFLD, although there are clinical trials ongoing with encouraging results.[34] Because the majority of patients

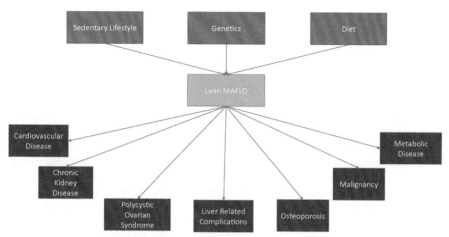

Fig. 2. Risk factors for, and complications of, lean MAFLD.

in these trials will be overweight/obese, the data may not specifically apply to the lean population. Hence, a key goal once the initial clinical trials have been completed is to undertake studies in other MAFLD subgroups, including those that are lean.

RESEARCH

At this time, there is limited published research into lean MAFLD as a standalone entity. Despite similar outcomes, and what appears to be a somewhat different pathophysiologic pathway to disease, the majority of studies have addressed lean MAFLD through subgroup analysis of data. Current research has been hampered by a lack of a standardized definition of lean MAFLD, which has led to further

---

Box 1
Open research questions on lean metabolic-associated fatty liver disease

Definition
• What is the standardized definition of lean MAFLD?
• Do diabetic patients with MAFLD of healthy weight fall within the criteria of lean MAFLD?
• Is BMI an appropriate measure to define lean MAFLD among ethnic groups?

Prevalence
• What is the global prevalence of lean MAFLD?
• What are the ethnic variations in lean MAFLD?

Pathophysiology
• What are the pathophysiologic differences between lean and nonlean MAFLD?
• What are the features that correspond with higher rates of hepatic and extrahepatic complications in lean MAFLD?
• Do noninvasive liver fibrosis scores in lean MAFLD correspond to that in the nonlean MAFLD population? If not, what noninvasive markers are needed to be developed that will allow clinicians to exclude significant fibrosis?
• Does lean MAFLD have the same levels of hepatic and extrahepatic complications when compared with the wider MAFLD population?

Treatment
• How effective are lifestyle interventions for lean MAFLD?
• How effective will pharmacotherapies be for lean MAFLD?

heterogeneity in published data. In addition, the utilization of nonobese MAFLD to encompass both lean and overweight MAFLD has hampered the generalizability of the published data.

Although the MAFLD diagnostic criterion has provided individuals with the ability to succinctly diagnose MAFLD in the community, there have been a number of maladaptive interpretations of lean MAFLD. Many studies have applied a stepwise strategy for MAFLD diagnosis, first identifying patients with type 2 diabetes followed by those who are overweight or obese, and then finally those with metabolic dysregulatory risk factors. Using this stepwise model, they have designated patients with diabetes MAFLD, overweight/obese MAFLD, and then lean MAFLD to represent those who only have metabolic dysregulatory risk factors. The diagnostic criterion was not intended to validate only 1 MAFLD phenotype at a time while discarding the others.[3] Thus, patients who have more than 1 MAFLD phenotype could potentially have additional risks of hepatic and extrahepatic complications and respond differently to management strategies and potential treatments. It is imperative that this be addressed sufficiently to provide enough granular detail regarding these patients, as subsets of MAFLD may need adjustments in screening, follow-up, and management based upon their disease cause (**Box 1**).

SUMMARY

Lean MAFLD is a clinical entity with similar rates of hepatic and extrahepatic complications to the wider MAFLD population. Because of the lower incidence of lean MAFLD, further research is needed to understand the prevalence, underlying pathophysiology, and management strategies applicable to this population of patients.

CLINICS CARE POINTS

- Metabolically unhealthy individuals can have "normal" weight and suffer from metabolic-associated fatty liver disease.
- Lean metabolic-associated fatty liver disease should be considered in patients with liver derangements or steatosis $\geq 5\%$ on imaging.
- With the new diagnostic criterion for metabolic-associated fatty liver disease, dual liver causes can be considered.
- Patients with lean metabolic-associated fatty liver disease should be assessed for extrahepatic complications, including cardiovascular and chronic kidney disease.
- Current management strategies for lean metabolic-associated fatty liver disease are diet and exercise, although there is limited evidence for their effectiveness.

DISCLOSURE

The authors have nothing to disclose.

REFERENCES

1. Ludwig J, Viggiano TR, McGill DB, Oh BJ. Nonalcoholic steatohepatitis: mayo clinic experiences with a hitherto unnamed disease. Mayo Clin Proc 1980; 55(7):434–8.
2. Shiha G, Korenjak M, Eskridge W, et al. Redefining fatty liver disease: an international patient perspective. Lancet Gastroenterol Hepatol 2021;6(1):73–9.

3. Eslam M, Newsome PN, Sarin SK, et al. A new definition for metabolic dysfunction-associated fatty liver disease: An international expert consensus statement. J Hepatol 2020;73(1):202–9.

4. Eslam M., El-Serag H.B., Francque S., et al., Metabolic (dysfunction)-associated fatty liver disease in individuals of normal weight, Nat Rev Gastroenterol Hepatol, 19 (10), 2022, 638–651.

5. Ye Q, Zou B, Yeo YH, et al. Global prevalence, incidence, and outcomes of non-obese or lean non-alcoholic fatty liver disease: a systematic review and meta-analysis. Lancet Gastroenterol Hepatol 2020;5(8):739–52.

6. Ordonez-Vazquez A.L., Juarez-Hernandez E., Zuarth-Vazquez J.M., et al., Impact on Prevalence of the Application of NAFLD/MAFLD Criteria in Overweight and Normal Weight Patients, Int J Environ Res Public Health, 19 (19), 2022, 12221.

7. Chan K.E., Koh T.J.L., Tang A.S.P., et al., Global Prevalence and Clinical Characteristics of Metabolic-associated Fatty Liver Disease: A Meta-Analysis and Systematic Review of 10 739 607 Individuals, J Clin Endocrinol Metab, 107 (9), 2022, 2691–2700.

8. Dao A.D., Nguyen V.H., Ito T., et al., Prevalence, characteristics, and mortality outcomes of obese and nonobese MAFLD in the United States, Hepatol Int, 17 (1), 2023, 225–236.

9. Guan C, Fu S, Zhen D, et al. Metabolic (Dysfunction)-Associated Fatty Liver Disease in Chinese Patients with Type 2 Diabetes from a Subcenter of the National Metabolic Management Center. J Diabetes Res 2022;2022:8429847.

10. Guan L., Zhang X., Tian H., et al., Prevalence and risk factors of metabolic-associated fatty liver disease during 2014-2018 from three cities of Liaoning Province: an epidemiological survey, BMJ Open, 12 (2), 2022, e047588.

11. Kim M., Yoon E.L., Cho S., et al., Prevalence of advanced hepatic fibrosis and co-morbidity in metabolic dysfunction-associated fatty liver disease in Korea, Liver Int, 42 (7), 2022, 1536–1544.

12. Lee H., Lim T.S., Kim S.U., et al., Long-term cardiovascular outcomes differ across metabolic dysfunction-associated fatty liver disease subtypes among middle-aged population, Hepatol Int, 16 (6), 2022, 1308–1317.

13. Yu C., Wang M., Zheng S., et al., Comparing the Diagnostic Criteria of MAFLD and NAFLD in the Chinese Population: A Population-based Prospective Cohort Study, J Clin Transl Hepatol, 10 (1), 2022, 6–16.

14. Yuan Q, Wang H, Gao P, et al. Prevalence and Risk Factors of Metabolic-Associated Fatty Liver Disease among 73,566 Individuals in Beijing, China. Int J Environ Res Public Health 2022;19(4).

15. Zeng J., Qin L., Jin Q., et al., Prevalence and characteristics of MAFLD in Chinese adults aged 40 years or older: A community-based study, Hepatobiliary Pancreat Dis Int, 21 (2), 2022, 154–161.

16. Cheng Y-M, Kao J-H, Wang C-C. The metabolic profiles and body composition of lean metabolic-associated fatty liver disease. Hepatology International 2021; 15(2):405–12.

17. Miao L., Yang L., Guo L.S., et al., Metabolic Dysfunction-associated Fatty Liver Disease is Associated with Greater Impairment of Lung Function than Nonalcoholic Fatty Liver Disease, J Clin Transl Hepatol, 10 (2), 2022, 230–237.

18. Sun DQ, Jin Y, Wang TY, et al. MAFLD and risk of CKD. Metabolism 2021;115: 154433.

19. Targher G, Tilg H, Byrne CD. Non-alcoholic fatty liver disease: a multisystem disease requiring a multidisciplinary and holistic approach. Lancet Gastroenterol Hepatol 2021;6(7):578–88.

20. Park H., Yoon E.L., Kim M., et al., Comparison of diagnostic performance between FIB-4 and NFS in metabolic-associated fatty liver disease era, *Hepatol Res*, 52 (3), 2022, 247–254.

21. Younes R., Govaere O., Petta S., et al., Caucasian lean subjects with non-alcoholic fatty liver disease share long-term prognosis of non-lean: time for reappraisal of BMI-driven approach?, *Gut*, 71 (2), 2022, 382–390.

22. Eren F, Kaya E, Yilmaz Y. Accuracy of Fibrosis-4 index and non-alcoholic fatty liver disease fibrosis scores in metabolic (dysfunction)-associated fatty liver disease according to body mass index: failure in the prediction of advanced fibrosis in lean and morbidly obese individuals. Eur J Gastroenterol Hepatol 2022;34(1):98–103.

23. Fu C., Wai J.W., Nik Mustapha N.R., et al., Performance of Simple Fibrosis Scores in Nonobese Patients With Nonalcoholic Fatty Liver Disease, *Clin Gastroenterol Hepatol*, 18 (12), 2020, 2843–2845.e2.

24. Mózes F.E., Lee J.A., Selvaraj E.A., et al., Diagnostic accuracy of non-invasive tests for advanced fibrosis in patients with NAFLD: an individual patient data meta-analysis, *Gut*, 71 (5), 2022, 1006–1019.

25. Liu Z, Suo C, Shi O, et al. The Health Impact of MAFLD, a Novel Disease Cluster of NAFLD, Is Amplified by the Integrated Effect of Fatty Liver Disease-Related Genetic Variants. Clin Gastroenterol Hepatol 2022;20(4):e855–75.

26. Chan W-K. Comparison between obese and non-obese NAFLD. Clinical and Molecular Hepatology 2022;107(9):2691–700.

27. Al-Omary A., Byth K., Weltman M., et al., The importance and impact of recognizing metabolic dysfunction-associated fatty liver disease in patients with chronic hepatitis C, *J Dig Dis*, 23 (1), 2022, 33–43.

28. Lin Y.-P., Lin S.-H., Wang C.-C., et al., Impact of MAFLD on HBV-Related Stage 0/A Hepatocellular Carcinoma after Curative Resection, *J Personalized Med*, 11 (8), 2021, 684.

29. Fukunaga S., Nakano D., Tsutsumi T., et al., Lean/normal-weight metabolic dysfunction-associated fatty liver disease is a risk factor for reflux esophagitis, *Hepatol Res*, 52 (8), 2022, 699–711.

30. Bessho R., Kashiwagi K., Ikura A., et al., A significant risk of metabolic dysfunction-associated fatty liver disease plus diabetes on subclinical atherosclerosis, *PLoS One*, 17 (5), 2022, e0269265.

31. Peng D, Yu Z, Wang M, et al. Association of Metabolic Dysfunction-Associated Fatty Liver Disease With Left Ventricular Diastolic Function and Cardiac Morphology. Front Endocrinol 2022;13:935390.

32. Chen X, Chen S, Pang J, et al. Are the different MAFLD subtypes based on the inclusion criteria correlated with all-cause mortality?, J Hepatol, 75(4), 2021, 987–989.

33. Semmler G, Wernly S, Bachmayer S, et al., Metabolic Dysfunction-Associated Fatty Liver Disease (MAFLD)-Rather a Bystander Than a Driver of Mortality, J Clin Endocrinol Metab, 106(9), 2021, 2670–2677.

34. Paternostro R, Trauner M. Current treatment of non-alcoholic fatty liver disease. J Intern Med 2022;292(2):190–204.

Lipid Disorders and Metabolic-Associated Fatty Liver Disease

Shima Dowla Anwar, MD, PhD[a], Christy Foster, MD[b],
Ambika Ashraf, MD[b],*

KEYWORDS

• MAFLD • NAFLD • Dyslipidemia • Statin • Fibrate • Eicosapent ethyl

KEY POINTS

- Lipotoxicity in the liver from the accumulation of free fatty acids and unesterified free cholesterol, defective very low-density lipoprotein export, excessive triglyceride deposition in the liver, abnormal metabolism of bile acids, and mitochondrial inflexibility are important factors in the etiopathogenesis of metabolic-associated fatty liver disease (MAFLD).
- Several genes (PNPLA3, TM6SF2, MBOAT7, HSD17B13, GCKR-P446 L) and some transcription factors (sterol regulatory element binding protein-2, farnesoid X receptor [FXR], and liver X receptor 9) that are involved in lipid metabolism can increase susceptibility for MAFLD.
- The management strategy usually involves lifestyle changes targeting body weight reduction $\geq$7%, and appropriate medical/surgical interventions aiming lipid-lowering and amelioration of cardiovascular disease risk.

INTRODUCTION

Metabolic-associated fatty liver disease (MAFLD) is now considered the most frequent cause of chronic liver disease in the world because of the alarming rise in obesity across the globe in the past few decades. MAFLD was named considering the systemic nature of the disease compared with the term nonalcoholic fatty liver disease (NAFLD) which represents the hepatic manifestation of the disease.[1] Recent data suggest that MAFLD now affects more than one-third of the global population with the prevalence estimates varying from region to region, and a steady and exponential increase in the epidemiologic trend reported globally regardless of the economic

[a] Department of Pediatrics, Boston Children Hospital, Harvard Medical School, Boston, MA, USA; [b] University of Alabama at Birmingham, 1601, 4th Avenue South, CPP M 30, Birmingham, AL 35233, USA
* Corresponding author.
E-mail address: AAshraf@uabmc.edu

Endocrinol Metab Clin N Am 52 (2023) 445–457
https://doi.org/10.1016/j.ecl.2023.01.003
0889-8529/23/© 2023 Elsevier Inc. All rights reserved.

endo.theclinics.com

status.[2] As MAFLD is usually a direct consequence of excess visceral adiposity related to physical inactivity and adverse dietary habits, several other metabolic-/obesity-related disorders such as dyslipidemia, type 2 diabetes mellitus (T2DM), metabolic syndrome, and hypertension often coexist along with substantial increase in the cardiovascular disease (CVD) risk.[3] Although MAFLD is mostly associated with visceral adiposity, patients with primary lipid disorders as well as those with generalized or acquired lipodystrophy can also develop the disease even in the absence of classic obesity.[4] In this evidence-based review, we elucidate the interlink between MAFLD and dyslipidemia to enable physicians to approach patients from the preventive and therapeutic perspectives.

Epidemiology

MAFLD is estimated to be the most common cause of liver disease in the United States and global estimates are between 20% and 45% in high-risk groups. It is more common in men and there is increased prevalence with older age. In children, the development of MAFLD is associated with higher risks of progression to cirrhosis, development of hepatocellular carcinoma, and requirement for transplantation.[5] The prevalence of MAFLD can be as high as 80% to 90% in adults with obesity, 70% in patients with obesity and diabetes,[6] and up to 90% in patients with hyperlipidemia.[7] The prevalence of MAFLD among children is 3% to 10%, rising to 40% to 70% among children with obesity. Moreover, pediatric MAFLD increased from about 3% a decade ago to 5% today, with a male-to-female ratio of 2:1.[7] There is a growing body of studies that examine the link between MAFLD and its association with atherogenic lipid profiles. Dyslipidemia, especially hypertriglyceridemia, can further increase the risk of MAFLD.

Primary Dyslipidemia

Patients with MAFLD exhibit atherogenic dyslipidemia characterized by the increased level of plasma triglycerides (TG), increased small dense low-density lipoprotein (LDL) particles, and decreased levels of high-density lipoprotein (HDL) particles.[8] Some of the genetic dyslipidemias can also be associated in some patients with MAFLD; a heterogeneous phenotype of disorders characterized by abnormal levels of circulating lipids and lipoproteins. These abnormalities include elevations in cholesterol, such as in familial hypercholesterolemia (isolated LDL cholesterol elevation or Fredrickson Class IIa), elevated TG (hypertriglyceridemia, Frederickson Classes I, IV, and V), or a combination of the two (Fredrickson Classes III or IIb)[9] as well as monoallelic mutations in ABHD5, involved in neutral lipid metabolism.[10]

Genetic Susceptibility

Ethnic variability has been noted in the development of MAFLD. Twin studies have shown that the heritability of MAFLD is approximately 50%.[11] Genome-wide studies have illustrated several key genetic loci which have been tied to the development of MALFD.[12] One such gene encodes patatin-like phospholipase domain-containing protein 3 (*PNPLA3*). Typically, this enzyme helps to hydrolyze TG by influencing the remodeling of fatty acid (FA) chains in liver TG, and therefore, a single nucleotide polymorphism (SNP) variant leads to the accumulation of TG in the hepatocytes. Carriage of the *PNPLA3-I148 M* variant will indicate a risk of a poorer prognosis of MAFLD.[12]

A specific polymorphism (rs58542926 A > G) in *TM6SF2* is associated with hepatic steatosis and progressive fibrosis. Mice studies have demonstrated that even with a normal diet, the *TM6SF2* knockout mice will develop hypercholesterolemia, elevated liver enzymes, and hepatic steatosis.[12]

The *MBOAT7* gene encodes lysophosphatidylinositol acyltransferase 1 which stimulates the incorporation of arachidonic acid into phosphatidylinositol leading to increased TG synthesis and accumulation in hepatocytes.[12]

In the liver, glucokinase regulatory protein (GKRP) regulates glucokinase activity. Initially, the *GCKR-P446 L* variant led to increased TG and hepatic steatosis.[12]

Hydroxysteroid 17-beta dehydrogenase 13 (*HSD17B13*) is a liver-specific, lipid droplet-associated protein, with retinol dehydrogenase activity. Its overexpression results in the development of steatosis in mice. Loss-of-function variants are protective against the development of nonalcoholic steatohepatitis (NASH).[12]

Cholesterol homeostasis is closely controlled by several nuclear transcription factors including sterol regulatory element binding protein (SREBP-2), FXR, and liver X receptor (LXR). SREBP-2 is a transcription factor which detects membrane cholesterol and FA content and will alter gene transcription involved in cholesterol synthesis. FXR is a nuclear receptor that detects bile acids and, in the liver, upregulates the uptake of HDL from circulation. FXR suppresses bile acid synthesis. It also promotes TG removal from hepatocytes and protects against hepatic steatosis. LXRs are nuclear cholesterol sensors that are activated by high levels of oxysterols. It will lead to increased cholesterol secretion from the body and increased LDL-receptor (LDLR) degradation.[13,14] Insulin resistance (IR) and compensatory hyperinsulinemia activate LXR and drive steatosis.

Secondary dyslipidemia
There are several different mechanisms for the development of secondary dyslipidemia. The most common cause is obesity. Obesity and IR increase the activity of hormone-sensitive lipase (HSL) which leads to increased lipolysis from the dysfunctional adipocytes and increased free FA (FFA) flux to the liver.[15] This FFA flux is compounded by the de novo lipogenesis (DNL) (from glucose and fructose) ultimately leading to hepatic steatosis. Moreover, excessive carbohydrate intake will lead to DNL in the liver. Hyperinsulinemia (secondary to IR) can lead to the upregulation of the key enzymes in lipogenesis.[16,17] Obesity is also associated with chronic inflammation which enhances the effects of lipotoxicity leading to the destruction of hepatocytes.

Conditions such as hypothyroidism, diabetes, and nephrotic syndrome can predispose to the development of MAFLD. Thyroid hormone will stimulate LDL hepatic uptake and degradation, and the production of bile acids by inducing LDLR expression. With hypothyroidism, the reduced/absent thyroid hormone will lead to a build-up of LDL cholesterol.[7] Thyroid hormone receptor (TR) β activation promotes hepatic FA uptake and mitochondrial oxidation.

The renal disease also can lead to dyslipidemia leading to MAFLD. Dyslipidemia can be due to urinary protein loss resulting in the overproduction of lipoproteins from the liver. Hepatic lipase (HL) and lipoprotein lipase (LPL) activity are both decreased in renal disease. Treatment with both a low-fat diet and pharmacotherapy such as fibrates and statins may be required in such patients.

Uncontrolled diabetes can lead to hyperchylomicronemia during times of diabetic ketoacidosis due to deficient activity of LPL, enhanced HSL, and reduced activity of endothelial lipase and HL.[16] IR will lead to enhanced HSL activity which hydrolyzes TG to FFA, which in turn will increase hepatic very low-density lipoprotein (VLDL) production, which is the predominant fasting plasma TG-carrying particle. IR will lead to decreased LPL activity which will impair VLDL clearance, promoting hypertriglyceridemia.

A few medications can also cause secondary dyslipidemia leading to MAFLD. The culprit drugs include steroids, estrogens, diuretics, and antitypical antipsychotics.

Steroids will increase hepatic VLDL production leading to elevated TG and LDL. Estrogens will increase VLDL production. Atypical antipsychotics predispose to obesity and IR, and thus, increased TG and reduced HDL levels.[18]

Natural History

MAFLD in most instances is a slowly progressive disease. There are multiple 'hits' proposed for progression from normal liver architecture to steatosis, and then to NASH.[13] The primary inciting factor is often IR which promotes the accumulation of neutral lipids within the hepatocytes leading to steatosis. Increased oxidation of fatty acids will lead to the production of reactive oxygen species (ROS), and thus, DNA damage, mitochondrial damage, and release of proinflammatory cytokines.[13] Previous studies indicate that around 25% of patients will progress to hepatitis and fibrosis. Progression to fibrosis is slow, over approximately 7 to 14 years depending on the level of hepatitis.[19] About 41% of patients with NASH will progress to fibrosis.[13] The extrahepatic manifestations such as complications related to IR and obesity (ie, hyperglycemia, diabetes, cardiac steatosis, subclinical inflammation) may regulate the disease progression.

Factors affecting disease progression

The gut microbiome has been identified as a significant contributor to the development of MAFLD. For example, an abundance of bacterial species, such as *Proteobacteria, Enterobacteria, Escherichia*, or *Bacteroides*, is observed in patients with NASH as compared with matched healthy individuals. The gut barrier was noted to be dysfunctional and more permeable in those with MAFLD. This increased permeability leads to enhanced translocation of lipopolysaccharide through the liver which can worsen liver inflammation. Dietary intake of fructose and glucose will be another significant contributor to the progression of MAFLD. Complex carbohydrates such as dietary fiber are protective against the progression as they are digested by the gut microbiome leading to the release of short-chain FA, which activate GPR43 signaling in adipose tissue and inhibit fat accumulation in the adipose tissue and liver.[20]

Pathobiological Interlink Between Metabolic-Associated Fatty Liver Disease and Dyslipidemia

MAFLD is often a histologic diagnosis and hence understanding the pathogenesis and pathophysiology is complicated. **Fig. 1** illustrates the link between dyslipidemia and

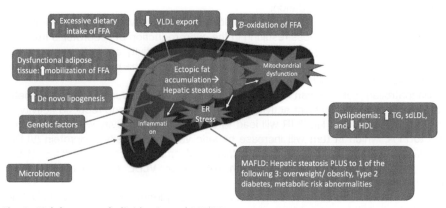

Fig. 1. Link between dyslipidemia and MAFLD.

MAFLD. The historical concept of pathogenesis is linked to IR and hepatic FFA accumulation causing steatosis. In this model, the initial event in the development of MAFLD could be the accumulation of FFA and subsequent excessive TG deposition in the liver. These lipids arise from three sources: (1) mobilization from adipocytes, (2) DNL from chronic nutritional overload and dysglycemia, and (3) excess dietary FFA.[13] There are two mechanisms of clearing FFA in the liver, namely beta-oxidation of FFA in the mitochondria and VLDL export. VLDL-TG hydrolysis depends on LPL and HL. Increased hepatic TG can lead to increased plasma TG by enhanced secretion from the liver. Hepatic steatosis will occur when the balance of TG synthesis and storage versus clearance is inadequate. This excess TG load coupled with increased DNL stimulates ROS and toxic lipid species (ceramides and diacylglycerides) leading to enhanced lipotoxicity.[21]

In addition to the above-described IR and FFA-centric pathogenic model, where the accumulation of neutral lipids causes MAFLD, recently it has been reported that accumulation of unesterified free cholesterol (FC) is also responsible for developing MAFLD.[13] The elevated intracellular cholesterol can inhibit the SREBP-2 pathway which in turn reduces LDL-receptor expression leading to reduced hepatic LDL uptake. Moreover, IR, a risk factor and key player in MAFLD pathogenesis, also influences bile acid metabolism. Indeed, FXR and TGR5 regulate glucose and lipid metabolism as well as inflammation, and thus, their pharmacologic agonists are proposed for the treatment of obesity, type 2 diabetes, and NASH. Excessive hepatic accumulation of neutral lipids, that is, FC is a critical component of MAFLD, which is driven by increased cholesterol esterification, attenuation of cholesterol export, and abnormal bile acid synthesis pathways.[14] Bile acids serve as metabolic modulators in the pathophysiology.

Oxidative and endoplasmic reticulum (ER) stress are the key factors which will contribute to the progression of hepatic fibrosis. In general, the mitochondria, ER, xanthine oxidase, and cytochrome P450 metabolism are the main sources of ROS.[22] Increased DNL reduces FA oxidation. Beta-oxidation is the main source of ROS in MAFLD. ROS will lead to a vicious cycle when they damage the electron transport chain. Both ROS and lipid peroxidation products will damage mitochondrial DNA. Excessive ROS will also lead to mitochondrial swelling and impaired mitochondrial cholesterol transport. This will sensitize hepatocytes to cytokine signaling contributing to cell death and apoptosis.[14] The mitochondrial 'inflexibility' is thought to be a major player in NASH.[23] FC accumulation in liver mitochondria induces lipotoxic mitochondrial dysfunction and increased oxidative stress leading to accelerated progression of MAFLD.[2,14]

ER has difficulty tolerating high lipid environments. Under stress conditions with FFA overload, the unfolded and misfolded proteins accumulate in the ER lumen. The cumulative response is to block the initiation of translation to reduce the load on the ER and when the damage is beyond repair, to induce apoptosis.[24] These changes will lead to a repetitive cycle. Liver injury and fibrogenesis are perpetrated through the activation of intracellular signaling in Kupffer cells, Stellate cells, and hepatocytes.

Clinical Evaluation

The diagnosis of MAFLD with concomitant dyslipidemia remains challenging as both conditions typically present asymptomatically, thereby, relying exclusively on health care providers for appropriate screening.[1] MAFLD is considered when there is the presence of hepatic steatosis (either by blood biomarker, histologic hepatic steatosis, or imaging evidence) along with at least one of the following three criteria: overweight/obesity, established T2D or presence of metabolic dysregulation. At least two of the following seven components need to be met to consider metabolic dysregulation: increased waist circumference, low HDL cholesterol, elevated TG for age and gender, hypertension, prediabetes, homeostatic model assessment (HOMA) IR score of ≥ 2.5, and high-sensitivity c-reactive protein (hsCRP) > 2 mg/L. There is currently no consensus among professional organizations regarding screening guidelines for MAFLD.[25] The American Association for the Study of Liver Diseases (AASLD), for example, recommends against routine screening, even in high-risk subgroups such as those with metabolic syndrome, obesity, and T2D, due to poor sensitivities of current screening modalities and lack of cost-effectiveness for early detection.[26] The European Association for the Study of the Liver, however, makes the opposite recommendation, that is, increasing routine screening of high-risk groups.[25] Nonetheless, before obtaining any screening tests, clinicians should screen for these conditions by taking a detailed history, and evaluating known risk factors, including race/ethnicity, family history, and comorbidities such as obesity, hypertension, and IR. This section discusses the traditional methods to screen for MAFLD and dyslipidemia.

Laboratory Testing

Diagnosis often begins with abnormal liver enzymes in a person with risk factors. Serum biomarkers for the evaluation of MAFLD/NASH include liver enzymes (alanine transaminase [ALT], aspartate transaminase [AST], gamma-glutamyl transferase [GGT]), markers of hepatocyte injury (C-reactive protein [CRP], tumor necrosis factor-α [TNF-α], cytokeratin-18), and markers of liver fibrosis (hyaluronic acid).[27] Given the pathophysiology, clinicians must also add a lipid panel to their screening laboratory tests. Traditionally, only liver transaminases, ALT and AST, have been routinely used for the initial screening and diagnosis of NAFLD. These biomarkers are not only inexpensive and widely available but elevations have also been shown to correlate with some degree of hepatocyte injury. However, there are significant challenges in their use to diagnose MAFLD. AST and ALT can be elevated due to hepatic and nonhepatic injury, or may not even be elevated in MAFLD.[28] Consequently, their sensitivity rate and specificity rate for diagnosing MAFLD is 45% and 85%, respectively.[29] Furthermore, there lacks consensus on what elevation in liver transaminases is considered abnormal. For these reasons, many professional organizations do not recommend their use in routine screening.[26]

Once the elevated liver enzymes are identified, a liver ultrasound is the next step. It is also essential to evaluate for associated diabetes (glycated hemoglobin; HbA1c) and dyslipidemia.

Other Diagnostic Modalities

Liver biopsy remains the gold standard method to prove steatosis, hepatitis, or fibrosis, but is least practical or feasible method, given its particularly invasive nature and the potential for complications. Several innovative imaging modalities have been developed to assess the degree of liver fibrosis. Dowla and colleagues have summarized the strengths and limitations of various imaging modalities for MAFLD.[30] Among all available modalities, the two that hold the most promise are MRI and ultrasonographic (US) elastography, both of which can differentiate between levels of fibrosis, although they differ in operator dependency and cost (with MRI being more expensive but less reliant on operator skill).

Complications

Dyslipidemia in patients with MAFLD presents as elevated TG or LDL cholesterol or reduced HDL cholesterol levels, all known to be important risk factors for the development of atherosclerosis, and consequently, CVD.[31] Specific CVD risk factors, such as carotid intima-media thickness, coronary artery calcification, elevated CRP levels, and high Framingham risk score are observed in patients with MAFLD, suggesting an inextricable link between the three diseases.[32] Therefore, it is not surprising that the leading cause of morbidity and mortality in this particular cohort is CVD.[33] Despite the strong association between MAFLD, dyslipidemia, and CVD, the complex mechanisms underlying their pathophysiology remain poorly understood. Studies suggest that local and systemic inflammation as well as oxidative stress caused by MAFLD create endothelial dysfunction, thereby, increasing the risk of CVD.[34] In particular, liver fat accumulation alongside oxidative stress releases inflammatory mediators (ie, TNF-α, CRP), increases expression of plasminogen activator inhibitor-1, and promotes endothelial dysfunction.[35] Therefore, therapeutic targets that both reduce excess hepatic lipid accumulation as well as attenuate the hepatic inflammatory response are ideal to combat the complications of MAFLD.

Management

Fig. 2 depicts the management algorithm.

Lifestyle Modification

Changes in diet and exercise, known as therapeutic lifestyle changes (TLC), are the mainstay of therapy for MAFLD. Consumption of a low carbohydrate diet has been shown to reduce plasma TG levels and improve insulin sensitivity despite not changing the body weight. Targeting ≥7% reduction of body weight if overweight or obese and limiting consumption of high fructose-containing beverages, and alcohol, and drinking ≥2 cups of caffeinated coffee daily are recommended.[36] A report from the AASLD, American College of Gastroenterology, and American Gastroenterological Association suggests that a gradual weight loss of 3% to 5% of one's body weight is recommended to improve hepatic steatosis; however, weight loss of 5% to 10% may be needed to reduce hepatic inflammation.[26] This degree of weight loss has been proven to resolve NASH in over 90% of patients.[37] Furthermore, recommendations for TLC are fairly nonspecific, including reduction of fat, sugar, and salt in the diet, use of a

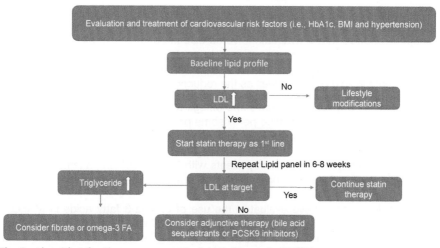

Fig. 2. Algorithm for the management of dyslipidemia in NAFLD.

hypocaloric diet, maintaining a body mass index [BMI] within normal limits, and exercising 30 to 60 minutes per day (preferably aerobic).

Medical Therapy

Given the link between the significant risk of CVD and MAFLD, it is essential to treat the associated dyslipidemia, which is usually characterized by atherogenic dyslipidemia with increased small-dense LDL, TG, and low HDL. However, it is important to keep in mind that the dysregulation of hepatic cholesterol homeostasis associated with MAFLD is not always associated with dyslipidemia. Several therapeutic agents, such as statins, fibrates, omega-3 FA, and insulin-sensitizing agents (metformin, thiazolidinediones) are being used depending on the clinical scenario.[38]

MAFLD is characterized by chronic hepatic steatosis. IR, a risk factor, and a key player in MAFLD pathogenesis, also influences lipid and bile acid metabolism. Conversely, bile acids fine-tune insulin responsiveness. Indeed, FXR and TGR5 regulate glucose and lipid metabolism, so that pharmacologic agonists are proposed for the treatment of obesity, T2DM, and NASH. It is essential to manage hyperglycemia and diabetes adequately. Several pharmacotherapies are being evaluated for NAFLD and NASH (ie, vitamin E, obeticholic acid) (FXR agonist), lanifibranor, firsocostat (inhibits DNL), resmetirom (THR-β agonist), etc.

Elevated plasma low-density lipoprotein: statins and low-density lipoprotein -lowering medications

Statins are the first line of treatment of elevated LDL. Statins are safe in MAFLD and have been shown to reduce the elevated liver enzymes in MAFLD.[39] Several statins are currently on the market, but some have received extra attention for their effects on improving MAFLD. Careful consideration for cardiovascular risk stratification should be given before determining when to initiate statin therapy. Studies suggest that MAFLD is associated with increased cardiovascular disease. Thus, pharmacotherapy needs to be considered depending on the associated risk factors. Risk factors such as hypertension, obesity/increased waist circumference, smoking, and family history of premature CVD are additional moderate risk factors that often coexist with the condition. Those patients with additional high-risk factors such as established CVD, or history of T2DM require a therapeutic goal of LDL <70 mg/dL.[40] Athyros and colleagues showed that 1600 patients with MAFLD treated with atorvastatin demonstrated significant improvement in TG, LDL, and total cholesterol, as well as a significant reduction in cardiovascular risk.[41] Similarly, in a small pilot study, Nelson and colleagues showed that simvastatin lowered LDL in patients with MAFLD after a 1-year follow-up period.[42] Finally, in a prospective cohort study, Antonopoulos and colleagues found that the MAFLD patients treated with rosuvastatin showed significant improvements in lipid profile as well as the reduction in total transaminases.[43]

Elevated plasma triglyceride: fibrates and omega-3 fatty acids

Fibrates reduce lipids by activating peroxisome proliferator-activated receptor alpha (PPARα), which increases lipolysis and facilitates fatty acid oxidation. Several studies have evaluated the effects of fibrates on MAFLD and have shown to improve the lipid profile and even hepatic function in patients with MAFLD.[44,45] In patients who have elevated serum TG, despite being on a statin, fibrates are helpful to reduce the CVD risk.[46]

Several clinical trials have evaluated the use of omega-3 fatty acids in MAFLD. Although these studies have mixed results on their effects on hepatic biomarkers, all have shown significant clinical evidence suggesting favorable improvement in TG in patients with NAFLD[47,48] Eicosapent ethyl (EPA) reduced the TG and reduced cardiovascular mortality. EPA inhibits the enzymes phosphatidic acid phosphatase and diacylglycerol acyltransferase which are involved in triglyceride synthesis. It also reduces TG levels by increasing VLDL and chylomicron clearance via lipoprotein lipase adherence.[49]

Fenofibrate and/or omega-3 fatty acid use should be considered if the fasting TG are greater than >500 mg/dL. Fibrates may also be added if fasting TG are between 200 and 499 mg/dL despite being on statin therapy.[40]

Insulin Sensitizers

As a fundamental component of MAFLD is IR, insulin sensitizers have a role in the management. Pioglitazones, semaglutide, and other glucagon-like peptide-1 (GLP-1) agonists have shown improvement in MAFLD and NASH. These are especially useful in patients with hyperglycemia and T2DM.

Surgical Treatment

The primary target of bariatric surgery for the treatment of MAFLD with dyslipidemia is weight loss. Weight loss following bariatric surgery has shown remarkably promising results. A meta-analysis evaluating the effect of bariatric surgery on MAFLD, including over 750 paired liver biopsies showed an improvement in hepatic fibrosis (65.5%), complete resolution of NASH (69.5%), improvement in steatohepatitis (81.3%), and improvement in steatosis (91.6%).[50] Those with improvements in metabolic profile and IR showed the most promising results.

Areas of Uncertainty/Emerging Concepts

Understanding the contribution of dyslipidemia to MAFLD is crucial. Factors related to hepatic steatosis and progression to MAFLD are well-known at this time. Insulin dysregulation and systemic response to metabolic overload are well-known aspects of the pathophysiology of MAFLD. The degree of obesity, caloric excess, magnitude of IR, and genetic predisposition to develop steatosis and oxidative damage are all critical elements to consider when designing management recommendations. Is there a specific window when the interventions are most effective? Traditionally IR and related hypertriglyceridemia is treated by caloric restriction and weight loss. Given the role of FC in hepatic inflammation, will reducing dietary cholesterol have an impact on steatosis and hepatotoxicity? There are no guidelines currently available that focus on treatment specific to the subtype of dyslipidemia seen in MAFLD.

The unavailability of adequate non-invasive specific biomarkers for screening of MAFLD poses a diagnostic challenge to clinicians. The current biochemical markers for screening of MAFLD such as ALT measurements are limited by inadequate specificity and sensitivity.

Other questions that need to be addressed are how to reduce fat and inflammation in the liver, reduce the lipotoxic load, and minimize lipotoxic injury to the mitochondria. There are unanswered aspects such as why some livers are more predisposed to MAFLD. There is a lot of heterogeneity in MAFLD. We do not fully know the signaling pathway issues. Can the inflammation be heightened by dyslipidemia and/or high cholesterol diet?

SUMMARY

MAFLD is a multifactorial, multisystemic disease which has become more prevalent. Dyslipidemia plays a key role in the etiopathogenesis of MAFLD along with abnormal transcription factors leading to oxidative stress and hepatocellular damage. Diagnosis involves laboratory evaluation and potential imaging. Screening for NAFLD by non-invasive measures and dyslipidemia in predisposed individuals may help in early detection. The current treatment options include lifestyle changes aiming at weight reduction, medications to treat dyslipidemia such as statin, fibrates, and eicosapent ethyl, management of diabetes, insulin sensitizers, and as well as bariatric surgery in certain cases. There are many open questions regarding the role of dyslipidemia in the pathoetiology and disease progression.

CLINICS CARE POINTS

- MAFLD, the most common cause of chronic liver disease in the world, is often associated with dyslipidemia which increases the CVD risk
- Both primary and secondary dyslipidemias can increase the risk of MAFLD and appropriate lipid-lowering therapy is crucial in the therapeutic algorithm of MAFLD to arrest the progression of the disease and CVD risk.
- Statins, fibrates, omega-3 fatty acids, bile acid sequestrants, and Proprotein convertase subtilisin/kexin type 9 (PCSK-9) inhibitors are all useful in the individualized medical management of dyslipidemia depending on the predominant biochemical and clinical characteristics of patients with MAFLD.

DISCLOSURE

No relevant disclosures to declare.

REFERENCES

1. Eslam M, Newsome P, Sarin S, et al. A new definition for metabolic dysfunction-associated fatty liver disease: an international expert consensus statement. J Hepatol 2020;73(1):202–9.
2. Le MH, Yeo Y, Xiaohe L, et al. 2019 Global NAFLD prevalence: a systematic review and meta-analysis. Clin Gastroenterol Hepatol 2022;20(12):2809–17, e28.
3. Yi M, Peng W, Feng F, et al. Extrahepatic morbidities and mortality of NAFLD: an umbrella review of meta-analyses. Aliment Pharmacol Ther 2022;56(7):1119–30.
4. Pirillo A, Casula M, Olmastroni E, et al. Global epidemiology of dyslipidaemias. Nat Rev Cardiol 2021;18(10):689–700.
5. Mitra S, De A, Chowdhury A. Epidemiology of non-alcoholic and alcoholic fatty liver diseases. Transl Gastroenterol Hepatol 2020;5:16.
6. Sunny NE, Bril F, Cusi K. Mitochondrial Adaptation in Nonalcoholic Fatty Liver Disease: Novel Mechanisms and Treatment Strategies. Trends Endocrinol Metab 2017;28(4):250–60.
7. Bellentani S, Scaglioni F, Marino M, et al. Epidemiology of non-alcoholic fatty liver disease. Dig Dis 2010;28(1):155–61.
8. Chatrath H, Vuppalanchi R, Chalasani N. Dyslipidemia in patients with nonalcoholic fatty liver disease. Semin Liver Dis 2012;32(1):22–9.
9. Patni N., Ahmad Z., Wilson D.P., Genetics and dyslipidemia, In: Feingold K.R., editor, Endotext. 2000, South; Dartmouth (MA). Bethesda, 1–21.
10. Youssefian L, Vahidnezhad H, Saeidian A, et al. Inherited non-alcoholic fatty liver disease and dyslipidemia due to monoallelic ABHD5 mutations. J Hepatol 2019; 71(2):366–70.

11. Loomba R, Schork N, Chen C, et al. Heritability of Hepatic Fibrosis and Steatosis Based on a Prospective Twin Study. Gastroenterology 2015;149(7):1784–93.

12. Martin K, Hatab A, Athwal V, et al. Genetic Contribution to Non-alcoholic Fatty Liver Disease and Prognostic Implications. Curr Diab Rep 2021;21(3):8.

13. Horn CL, Morales A, Savard C, et al. Role of Cholesterol-Associated Steatohepatitis in the Development of NASH. Hepatol Commun 2022;6(1):12–35.

14. Arguello G, Balboa E, Arrese M, et al. Recent insights on the role of cholesterol in non-alcoholic fatty liver disease. Biochim Biophys Acta 2015;1852(9):1765–78.

15. Fabbrini E, Sullivan S, Klein S. Obesity and nonalcoholic fatty liver disease: biochemical, metabolic, and clinical implications. Hepatology 2010;51(2): 679–89.

16. Hirano T. Pathophysiology of Diabetic Dyslipidemia. J Atheroscler Thromb 2018; 25(9):771–82.

17. Kitade H, Guanliang C, Ni Y, et al. Nonalcoholic Fatty Liver Disease and Insulin Resistance: New Insights and Potential New Treatments. Nutrients 2017;9(4):387.

18. Yanai H, Yoshida H. Secondary dyslipidemia: its treatments and association with atherosclerosis. Glob Health Med 2021;3(1):15–23.

19. Pais R, Maurel T. Natural History of NAFLD. J Clin Med 2021;10(6):1161.

20. Kolodziejczyk AA, Zheng D, Shibolet O, et al. The role of the microbiome in NAFLD and NASH. EMBO Mol Med 2019;11(2):e9302.

21. Yamaguchi K, Yang L, McCall S, et al. Inhibiting triglyceride synthesis improves hepatic steatosis but exacerbates liver damage and fibrosis in obese mice with nonalcoholic steatohepatitis. Hepatology 2007;45(6):1366–74.

22. Rolo AP, Teodoro JS, Palmeira CM. Role of oxidative stress in the pathogenesis of nonalcoholic steatohepatitis. Free Radic Biol Med 2012;52(1):59–69.

23. Koliaki C, Roden M. Hepatic energy metabolism in human diabetes mellitus, obesity and non-alcoholic fatty liver disease. Mol Cell Endocrinol 2013; 379(1–2):35–42.

24. Song B, Scheuner D, Ron D, et al. Chop deletion reduces oxidative stress, improves beta cell function, and promotes cell survival in multiple mouse models of diabetes. J Clin Invest 2008;118(10):3378–89.

25. Pandyarajan V, Gish R, Alkhouri N, Gish R, Alkhouri N, et al. Screening for Nonalcoholic Fatty Liver Disease in the Primary Care Clinic. Gastroenterol Hepatol 2019;15(7):357–65.

26. Chalasani N, Younossi Z, Lavine J, et al. The diagnosis and management of nonalcoholic fatty liver disease: Practice guidance from the American Association for the Study of Liver Diseases. Hepatology 2018;67(1):328–57.

27. Hyysalo J, Mannisto V, Zhou Y, et al. A population-based study on the prevalence of NASH using scores validated against liver histology. J Hepatol 2014;60(4): 839–46.

28. Mofrad P, Contos M, Haque M, et al. Clinical and histologic spectrum of nonalcoholic fatty liver disease associated with normal ALT values. Hepatology 2003; 37(6):1286–92.

29. Rinella ME. Nonalcoholic fatty liver disease: a systematic review. JAMA 2015; 313(22):2263–73.

30. Dowla S GA, Ashraf AP. Non-alcoholic fatty liver disease in children with obesity. In: Bagchi ID, editor. Global perspectives on childhood obesity: current status consequences and prevention. London: Elsevier/Academic Press; 2019. p. 255–65.

31. Sahebkar A, Chew GT, Watts GF. New peroxisome proliferator-activated receptor agonists: potential treatments for atherogenic dyslipidemia and non-alcoholic fatty liver disease. Expert Opin Pharmacother 2014;15(4):493–503.
32. Speliotes EK, Massaro J, Hoffmann U, et al. Fatty liver is associated with dyslipidemia and dysglycemia independent of visceral fat: the Framingham Heart Study. Hepatology 2010;51(6):1979–87.
33. Soderberg C, Stal P, Askling J, et al. Decreased survival of subjects with elevated liver function tests during a 28-year follow-up. Hepatology 2010; 51(2):595–602.
34. Liu H, Lu HY. Nonalcoholic fatty liver disease and cardiovascular disease. World J Gastroenterol 2014;20(26):8407–15.
35. Gaggini M, Morelli M, Buzzigoli E, et al. Non-alcoholic fatty liver disease (NAFLD) and its connection with insulin resistance, dyslipidemia, atherosclerosis and coronary heart disease. Nutrients 2013;5(5):1544–60.
36. Diehl AM, Day C. Cause, Pathogenesis, and Treatment of Nonalcoholic Steatohepatitis. N Engl J Med 2017;377(21):2063–72.
37. Vilar-Gomez E, Martinez-Perez Y, Calzadilla-Bertot L, et al. Weight Loss Through Lifestyle Modification Significantly Reduces Features of Nonalcoholic Steatohepatitis. Gastroenterology 2015;149(2):367–78, e5; quiz e14-5.
38. Zhang QQ, Lu LG. Nonalcoholic Fatty Liver Disease: Dyslipidemia, Risk for Cardiovascular Complications, and Treatment Strategy. J Clin Transl Hepatol 2015; 3(1):78–84.
39. Bril F, Portillo Sanchez P, Lomonaco R, et al. Liver Safety of Statins in Prediabetes or T2DM and Nonalcoholic Steatohepatitis: Post Hoc Analysis of a Randomized Trial. J Clin Endocrinol Metab 2017;102(8):2950–61.
40. Martin A, Lang S, Goeser T, et al. Management of Dyslipidemia in Patients with Non-Alcoholic Fatty Liver Disease. Curr Atheroscler Rep 2022;24(7):533–46.
41. Athyros VG, Tziomalos K, Gossios T, et al. Safety and efficacy of long-term statin treatment for cardiovascular events in patients with coronary heart disease and abnormal liver tests in the Greek Atorvastatin and Coronary Heart Disease Evaluation (GREACE) Study: a post-hoc analysis. Lancet 2010; 376(9756):1916–22.
42. Nelson A, Torres D, Morgan A, et al. A pilot study using simvastatin in the treatment of nonalcoholic steatohepatitis: A randomized placebo-controlled trial. J Clin Gastroenterol 2009;43(10):990–4.
43. Antonopoulos S, Mikros S, Mylonopoulou M, et al. Rosuvastatin as a novel treatment of non-alcoholic fatty liver disease in hyperlipidemic patients. Atherosclerosis 2006;184(1):233–4.
44. Athyros VG, Mikhailidis DP, Didangelos TP, et al. Effect of multifactorial treatment on non-alcoholic fatty liver disease in metabolic syndrome: a randomised study. Curr Med Res Opin 2006;22(5):873–83.
45. Fernandez-Miranda C, Perez-Carreras M, Lopez-Alonso G, et al. A pilot trial of fenofibrate for the treatment of non-alcoholic fatty liver disease. Dig Liver Dis 2008; 40(3):200–5.
46. Ginsberg H, Elam M, Lovato L, et al. Effects of combination lipid therapy in type 2 diabetes mellitus. N Engl J Med 2010;362(17):1563–74.
47. Capanni M, Calella F, Biagini MR, Genise S, et al. Prolonged n-3 polyunsaturated fatty acid supplementation ameliorates hepatic steatosis in patients with non-alcoholic fatty liver disease: a pilot study. Aliment Pharmacol Ther 2006;23(8): 1143–51.

48. Spadaro L, Magliocco O, Spampinato D, et al. Effects of n-3 polyunsaturated fatty acids in subjects with nonalcoholic fatty liver disease. Dig Liver Dis 2008;40(3): 194–9.
49. Bhatt DL, Steg PG, MIller M, et al. Cardiovascular Risk Reduction with Icosapent Ethyl for Hypertriglyceridemia. N Engl J Med 2019;380(1):11–22.
50. Mummadi RR, Kasturi KS, Chennareddygari S, et al. Effect of bariatric surgery on nonalcoholic fatty liver disease: systematic review and meta-analysis. Clin Gastroenterol Hepatol 2008;6(12):1396–402.

Cardiovascular Implications of Metabolic Dysfunction-Associated Fatty Liver Disease

Zhewen Ren, MS[a,b,c], Anke Wesselius, PhD[d,e],
Coen D.A. Stehouwer, MD, PhD[a,f],
Martijn C.G.J. Brouwers, MD, PhD[a,b],*

KEYWORDS

- Metabolic dysfunction-associated fatty liver disease
- Nonalcoholic fatty liver disease • Cardiovascular disease • Preventive measures
- Treatment

KEY POINTS

- Epidemiological studies have shown that both nonalcoholic fatty liver disease (NAFLD) and metabolic dysfunction-associated fatty liver disease (MAFLD) are associated with cardiovascular disease (CVD).
- Mendelian randomization studies have inferred a causal relationship between NAFLD/MAFLD and CVD.
- It is suggested that NAFLD/MAFLD is regarded as "high-risk" similar to diabetes, which justifies intensive lipid and blood pressure lowering therapy.
- Further studies are needed to elucidate the role of specific NAFLD/MAFLD stages in the pathogenesis of CVD.

INTRODUCTION

Nonalcoholic fatty liver disease (NAFLD) is currently the most common cause of chronic liver disease worldwide, with an estimated global prevalence of 32.4%.[1] Although

[a] Division of Endocrinology and Metabolic Disease, Department of Internal Medicine, Maastricht University Medical Center, P Debyelaan 25, 6229 HX Maastricht, the Netherlands; [b] CARIM School for Cardiovascular Diseases, Maastricht University, Universiteitssingel 50, 6229 ER Maastricht, the Netherlands; [c] Laboratory for Metabolism and Vascular Medicine, Maastricht University, Universiteitssingel 50, 6229 ER Maastricht, the Netherlands; [d] Department of Epidemiology, Maastricht University, Universiteitssingel 50, 6229 ER Maastricht, the Netherlands; [e] NUTRIM School for Nutrition and Translational Research in Metabolism Maastricht University, Universiteitssingel 50, 6229 ER Maastricht, the Netherlands; [f] Division of General Internal Medicine, Department of Internal Medicine, Maastricht University Medical Centre, P Debyelaan 25, 6229 HX Maastricht, the Netherlands
* Corresponding author.Division of Endocrinology and Metabolic Disease, Department of Internal Medicine, Maastricht University Medical Center, P Debyelaan 25, 6229 HX Maastricht.
E-mail address: mcgj.brouwers@mumc.nl

Endocrinol Metab Clin N Am 52 (2023) 459–468
https://doi.org/10.1016/j.ecl.2023.01.002
0889-8529/23/© 2023 Elsevier Inc. All rights reserved.

NAFLD has emerged as the principal reason for liver transplantation,[2] most patients with NAFLD die from cardiovascular disease (CVD).[3]

Recently, a group of international experts proposed to redefine NAFLD—originally diagnosed histologically as steatosis, nonalcoholic steatohepatitis (NASH), or fibrosis in the absence of excess alcohol consumption[4]—to metabolic dysfunction-associated fatty liver disease (MAFLD), which is defined as steatosis associated with either over-weight, diabetes, and/or a combination of other metabolic risk factors (ie, hyperten-sion, dyslipidemia, prediabetes, and insulin resistance).[5] The main purpose of the change was to make it an inclusive diagnosis prioritizing metabolic abnormalities.[5]

Both NAFLD and MAFLD are associated with many cardiovascular risk factors, such as dyslipidemia, insulin resistance, and hypertension.[6–8] The aim of the present review is to provide a comprehensive overview and interpretation of the existing literature on the association between NAFLD/MAFLD and CVD, and to provide physicians practical tools in order to prevent CVD in patients with NAFLD/MAFLD.

EPIDEMIOLOGICAL EVIDENCE

Observational studies have shown that NAFLD is associated with an increased risk of fatal or nonfatal CVD events. A recent meta-analysis by Mantovani and colleagues[9] based on 36 observational studies with a median follow-up duration of 6.5 years involving 5,802,226 middle-aged individuals, demonstrated that patients with NAFLD had a 45% higher risk (hazard ratio [HR]: 1.45; 95% confidence interval [CI]: 1.31–1.61) of developing fatal or nonfatal cardiovascular (CV) events (ie, myocardial infarction, ischemic/hemorrhagic stroke, coronary revascularizations, unstable angina, heart fail-ure, and CV death) in comparison to those without NAFLD. This risk was independent of common cardiometabolic risk factors such as body mass index, diabetes, hyper-tension, and dyslipidemia.

The risk of incident CVD seems to increase in parallel with NAFLD severity. In their meta-analysis, Mantovani and colleagues[9] concluded that CVD risk is particularly high in patients with advanced fibrosis (HR: 2.50; 95% CI: 1.68–3.72). Similar findings were recently observed in a Swedish cohort study, including 10,422 patients with biopsy-proven NAFLD who were followed for an average duration of 13.6 years. The minimally adjusted risk of major cardiovascular events (defined as ischemic heart disease, congestive heart failure, stroke, and cardiovascular mortality) was 1.80 (95%CI: 1.73–1.88), which increased from simple steatosis (HR: 1.74; 95% CI: 1.65–1.83), to NASH (HR: 1.81; 95% CI: 1.59–2.07), to fibrosis (HR: 1.93; 95% CI: 1.71–2.17), to cirrhosis (HR: 2.57; 95% CI: 2.16–3.04).[10]

Other observational studies have also provided evidence linking MAFLD to CVD. According to a recent meta-analysis based on 7 cohort studies involving 13,318,377 middle-aged individuals, individuals with MAFLD had a significantly greater risk of CVD than those without MAFLD (HR: 1.50; 95%CI: 1.30–1.72).[11] Although this risk es-timate was numerically higher than the risk observed for patients with NAFLD (HR: 1.27; 95%CI: 1.12–1.45), it was not significantly different statistically ($P = .097$).[11] It should, however, be noted that the diagnosis of both MAFLD and NAFLD was based on surrogate markers, such as the fatty liver index and the K-NAFLD score, in 4 of the included studies.[11] Because these indices are based on metabolic factors (such as waist circumference and serum triglycerides[12,13]), the definitions of MAFLD and NAFLD in these studies are much alike and, hence, may have mitigated any difference in the cardiovascular risk estimates between NAFLD and MAFLD.

Regardless of any difference between NAFLD and MAFLD, these studies clearly show that both entities are associated with an increased CVD risk. It can, however, not be concluded that NAFLD and MAFLD play a causal role in the pathogenesis of CVD. Although most studies adjusted for potential confounders, such age, sex, lifestyle factors, and serum lipids (which in fact is more likely a mediator than a confounder), residual confounding cannot be excluded.

EVIDENCE FOR A CAUSAL RELATIONSHIP

Mendelian randomization (MR) is a suitable approach to infer causality especially in chronic diseases.[14] In the absence of an extensive set of NAFLD-associated genes, the first studies focused on one gene variant as an instrumental variable. These studies demonstrated that a variant in the transmembrane 6 superfamily member 2 gene (TM6SF2)—which predisposes to NAFLD through an impaired very-low-density lipoprotein (VLDL) secretion—protects from coronary artery disease (CAD).[15,16] Similarly, a common variant in the patatin-like phospholipase domain-containing protein 3 gene (PNPLA3)—the first and most robustly reported NAFLD susceptibility gene[17]—also seemed to protect from CAD.[16] Although the exact function of PNPLA3 remains to be elucidated, stable isotope studies have shown that carriers of this common variant are also characterized by an impaired VLDL secretion.[18] In contrast to the findings for TM6F2 and PNPLA3, a meta-analysis showed that a common variant in GCKR—which has been associated with de novo lipogenesis and NAFLD[19,20]—predisposes to CAD.[21] More recently, similar findings have been observed for other de novo lipogenesis-associated genes.[22]

When more NAFLD susceptibility genes were identified, they were also clustered to study the association with CAD. However, no association was found.[23] Strikingly, exclusion of gene variants that predispose to NAFLD via an impaired VLDL secretion (such as PNPLA3 and TM6SF2) resulted in a positive association with CAD, whereas an inverse association was found for the cluster of VLDL secretion genes only.[23] Furthermore, when the associations of all NAFLD genes with CAD were plotted against their associations with serum lipids, a strong relationship was observed (**Fig. 1**). Of interest, the intercept of the regression line was zero, indicating that when a NAFLD susceptibility gene is not associated with serum lipids, there is also no relationship with CAD (see **Fig. 1**).[23] The interpretation of these genetic findings is severalfold: (1) the relationship between NAFLD and CAD depends on the underlying pathway that drives NAFLD, that is, an impaired VLDL production protects from CAD, whereas enhanced de novo lipogenesis predisposes to CAD, (2) the relationship between NAFLD and CAD seems to be mediated by serum lipids (see **Fig. 1**), and (3) other potential mediators, such as low-grade inflammation, seem to play only a minor role. Because many of the included gene variants (including PNPLA3, TM6SF2, and GCKR) are not only associated with simple steatosis but also with more advanced stages of NAFLD, it would have been expected that any NASH or fibrosis-mediated effect on CAD would have shifted the regression line upwards, that is, when there is no association with serum lipids, there is still a relationship with CAD (see **Fig. 1**).

Lauridsen and colleagues were the first to perform a MR study using PNPLA3 as an instrumental variable. They showed that genetically predicted NAFLD was not associated with ischemic heart disease (odds ratio [OR]: 0.98; 95%CI: 0.94–1.03) and, hence, concluded that the previously reported associations between NAFLD and CVD were likely explained by confounding.[24] It can, however, be argued whether PNPLA3 is a valid instrument for NAFLD in MR studies. First, the association between the common variant in PNPLA3 and impairment of VLDL secretion has both upstream and downstream effects, that is, accumulation of intrahepatic lipids and lowering of serum lipids (a well-reported protective factor for CVD), respectively. This is an

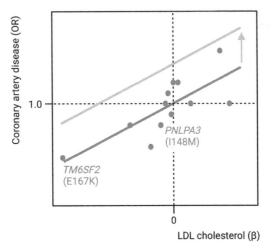

Fig. 1. Relationship between LDL cholesterol and risk of CAD conferred by NAFLD suscepti-bility genes (such as *TM6SF2* and *PNPLA3*). When a NAFLD susceptibility gene is not associ-ated with LDL cholesterol, there is also no association with CAD risk (regression line, *blue*). It would have been expected that the presence of other mediators, for example, low-grade inflammation, would have shifted the regression line upward (regression line, *gray*). CAD, coronary artery disease; LDL, low-density lipoprotein; NAFLD, nonalcoholic fatty liver dis-ease; OR, odds ratio; PNPLA3, patatin-like phospholipase domain-containing protein 3; TM6SF2, transmembrane 6 superfamily member 2. (Created with BioRender.com.)

example of horizontal pleiotropy, which violates the MR assumptions (**Fig. 2**). Second, it has been well established that an average patient with NAFLD is characterized by *increased* rather than *decreased* VLDL secretion.[25] The variant in *PNPLA3*, therefore, does not reflect the predominant pathways that result in NAFLD.

Very recently, the summarized data from large-scale genome-wide association studies for NAFLD have become publicly available,[26] which allowed the performance

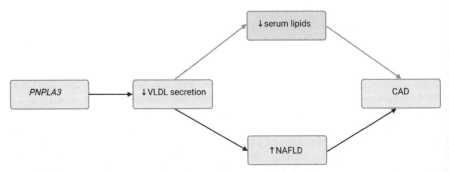

Fig. 2. The common variant in *PNPLA3* predisposes to NAFLD trough impaired VLDL secre-tion. Because impairment of VLDL secretion also results in lower serum lipids, there is hor-izontal pleiotropy *(grey pathway)* when the variant in *PNPLA3* is used as an instrumental variable to study the relationship between NAFLD and CAD *(blue pathway)*. Created with Biorender.com. CAD, coronary artery disease; NAFLD, nonalcoholic fatty liver disease; VLDL, very-low-density lipoprotein.

of 2-sample MR studies using an extensive set of NAFLD susceptibility genes as instrumental variables. We showed that—after exclusion of gene variants associated with impairment of VLDL secretion, for hitherto explained arguments—genetically predicted NAFLD was robustly associated with CAD (OR: 1.15; 95%CI: 1.04–1.28).[27]

These findings corroborate and extend the previously described results obtained from epidemiological studies because they suggest that the relationship between NAFLD and CAD is truly causal. The central role for simple steatosis, however, seems to be in conflict with the observational biopsy data, which pinpointed a prominent role for advanced NAFLD stages in CVD risk.[10] These epidemiological studies may be biased by differences in exposure time, that is, patients with advanced NAFLD stages may have a longer history of liver disease and, hence, a longer arterial wall exposure to atherogenic lipids in comparison to individuals with simple steatosis. Alternatively, it could be that advanced stages of NAFLD were underrepresented in the gene-CAD datasets used for the MR studies, which would explain why the intercept of the regression line in **Fig. 1** is zero.

IMPLICATIONS FOR TREATMENT OF NONALCOHOLIC FATTY LIVER DISEASE AND METABOLIC DYSFUNCTION-ASSOCIATED FATTY LIVER DISEASE

NAFLD/MAFLD treatment should ideally also have beneficial effects on CVD risk. Lifestyle intervention is the cornerstone of NAFLD/MAFLD treatment. Although weight reduction by means of diet, exercise and behavioral changes has been shown to reduce steatosis and NASH,[28] the effect on CVD risk is less straightforward. A relatively small (n = 537) but long-term follow-up study (23 years) showed that a 6-year lifestyle intervention program reduced the incidence of CVD.[29] In contrast, the Look AHEAD (Action for Health in Diabetes) study did not show any benefit of intensive lifestyle intervention on CVD outcomes (n = 5145; median follow-up: 9.6 years).[30] Of note, the use of statins and antihypertensive medications, which was higher in the usual care group,[30] may have mitigated any difference in incident CVD between both groups. Furthermore, a post hoc analysis showed a statistically significant reduction of CVD in those individuals who lost more than 10% body weight.[31] The benefits of large weight loss have also been reported by bariatric surgery, which results in resolution of all NAFLD stages, including fibrosis,[32] and a decrease in CVD death.[33]

Glucagon-like peptide-1 receptor (GLP-1R) agonists and pioglitazone are currently the only pharmacotherapeutic agents that have been shown to reduce both NASH and major adverse cardiovascular events.[34–41] They are, however, not yet approved by the US Food and Drug Administration or the European Medicines Agency for NAFLD/MAFLD treatment. Furthermore, the clinical applicability for pioglitazone is limited, given the propensity for several undesired side effects, including weight gain, heart failure, and fractures.[39] Of note, because these compounds are indicated for treatment of type 2 diabetes (T2D), they should be considered as part of tailored therapy in patients with T2D who are also affected by NAFLD/MAFLD.

IMPLICATIONS FOR PREVENTION OF CARDIOVASCULAR DISEASE

It seems rational that patients with NAFLD/MAFLD are screened for cardiometabolic risk factors, including hypertension, dyslipidemia, and T2D. This has indeed been endorsed by the European Association for the Study of Diabetes/European Association for the Study of the Liver/European Association for the Study of Obesity, the American Gastroenterological Association (AGA), and the American Association of Clinical Endocrinology Clinical Practice (co-sponsored by the American Association for the Study of Liver Disease).[42–44] It is, however, unclear which lipid and blood pressure treatment targets should be aimed for in primary prevention. Although the AGA recommends to perform risk stratification by estimating an individual's 10-year absolute atherosclerotic CVD (ASCVD) risk,[43] it is not yet clear whether current risk calculators (such as the ASCVD risk estimator, Framingham risk score, and the Systematic Coronary Risk Evaluation [SCORE])[45] accurately predict CVD risk in patients with NAFLD/MAFLD. Because these risk estimators have been developed in an era when preventive measures were not widely available, it is difficult to position NAFLD/MAFLD by performing studies in the modern era of widespread preventive measures. Such studies will tend to underestimate the true risk, as we have previously shown in dyslipidemic pedigrees enriched with NAFLD.[46]

Based on our previous MR studies—suggesting that serum lipids are the principal mediator of CVD risk in NAFLD (see **Fig. 1**)[23]—it could be argued that current risk estimators, which include serum lipids, should be sufficiently accurate. However, it could also be argued that NAFLD deserves the same status as T2D in CVD risk estimation because both traditional epidemiology and MR studies have shown that the CVD risk conferred by NAFLD is in the same order of magnitude as the CVD risk conferred by T2D.[10,27,47,48] This is further supported by the current MAFLD definition, which includes T2D.

The American College of Cardiology (ACC) and American Heart Association (AHA) recommend to prescribe high-intensity statin therapy to reduce LDL cholesterol levels by more than 50% in patients with diabetes,[45] whereas the European Society of Cardiology (ESC) advices to consider patients with diabetes as high-risk patients and to reduce LDL cholesterol to less than 2.6 mmol/L (<100 mg/dL) or even to less than 1.8 mmol/L (<70 mg/dL) depending on residual risk.[49] Because these targets are nowadays relatively easy to reach at low costs, thanks to potent, off-patent statins, we recommend to apply similar targets for NAFLD/MAFLD. Statin treatment is considered safe in NAFLD[50] and can be prescribed when serum transaminases are less than 3 times the upper limit of normal (provided liver function is normal).[51]

For blood pressure, the AHA/ACC guideline recommends to treat less than 130/80 mm Hg in diabetes,[45] whereas the ESC advices to lower systolic blood pressure

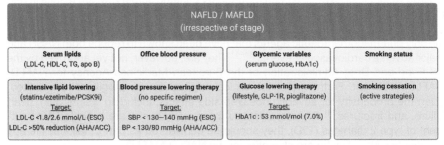

Fig. 3. Cardiovascular risk evaluation and management algorithm in patients with NAFLD/MAFLD. Cardiovascular risk evaluation should include serum lipids (apo B may be considered), office blood pressure, glycemic variables, and smoking status. Management consists of intensive lipid lowering, blood pressure lowering therapy, glucose lowering therapy (in case of T2D; preferably with interventions that have proven benefit on both NAFLD and CVD risk; the potential benefits of pioglitazone should be carefully weighed against the risks) and active smoking cessation strategies. Created with Biorender.com. AHA/ACC, American Heart Association/American College of Cardiology; apo B, apolipoprotein B; BP, blood pressure; ESC, European Society of Cardiology; GLP-1R, GLP-1 receptor agonist; HDL-C, HDL cholesterol; LDL-C, LDL cholesterol; PCSK9i, PCSK9 inhibitor; SBP, systolic blood pressure; TG, triglycerides.

to less than 140 mm Hg or even to less than 130 mm Hg depending on residual risk.[49]

AREAS OF UNCERTAINTY/EMERGING CONCEPTS

Besides the absence of evidence on how to position NAFLD/MAFLD in current cardiovascular risk estimation scores, it is also unclear whether the NAFLD/MAFLD stage matters. Stable isotope studies have shown that intrahepatic lipid accumulation, the first stage of NAFLD/MAFLD, is associated with the production of atherogenic lipid particles,[25] whereas epidemiological studies have assigned a role for advanced NAFLD stages.[9,52] Further studies are needed to unravel the involvement of the specific NAFLD/MAFLD stages and to identify their mediators in the pathogenesis of CVD.

Fig. 3 shows a cardiovascular risk evaluation and management algorithm in patients with NAFLD/MAFLD, based on current evidence.

SUMMARY

Both NAFLD and MAFLD are causally associated with CVD, which supports current guidelines to screen for cardiovascular risk factors in patients with NAFLD/MAFLD. It is suggested that NAFLD/MAFLD is regarded as "high-risk" similar to diabetes, which justifies intensive lipid and blood pressure lowering therapy.

CLINICS CARE POINTS

- NAFLD/MAFLD is established as a serious CVD risk factor comparable to the CVD risk associated with diabetes mellitus based on epidemiological and MR studies.

- Although there are some suggestions for higher risk of CVD in advanced stages NAFLD/MAFLD compared with simple steatosis based on current epidemiological data, more studies are required to establish the causal link for making firm recommendations regarding intensive risk reduction measures.

- Intense lifestyle, pharmacological and bariatric interventions aiming significant weight reduction, and adequate lipid lowering along with optimal blood pressure control are expected to reduce the CVD risk associated with NAFLD/MAFLD.

- It is advised to screen for cardiovascular risk factors in patients with NAFLD/MAFLD.

- It is suggested to regard NAFLD/MAFLD as high-risk, analogous to T2D, and to initiate intensive lipid-lowering and blood pressure-lowering therapy.

DECLARATION OF INTERESTS

The authors have nothing to disclose.

REFERENCES

1. Riazi K, Azhari H, Charette JH, et al. The prevalence and incidence of NAFLD worldwide: a systematic review and meta-analysis. The Lancet Gastroenterology & Hepatology 2022;7(9):851–61.
2. Younossi ZM, Stepanova M, Ong J, et al. Nonalcoholic Steatohepatitis Is the Most Rapidly Increasing Indication for Liver Transplantation in the United States. Clin Gastroenterol Hepatol 2021;19(3):580–9.e585.
3. Mantovani A, Scorletti E, Mosca A, et al. Complications, morbidity and mortality of nonalcoholic fatty liver disease. Metab Clin Exp 2020;111s:154170.

4. Ludwig J, Viggiano TR, McGill DB, et al. Nonalcoholic steatohepatitis: mayo clinic experiences with a hitherto unnamed disease. Mayo Clin Proc 1980;55(7):434–8.

5. Eslam M, Newsome PN, Sarin SK, et al. A new definition for metabolic dysfunction-associated fatty liver disease: An international expert consensus statement. J Hepatol 2020;73(1):202–9.

6. Dongiovanni P, Paolini E, Corsini A, et al. Nonalcoholic fatty liver disease or metabolic dysfunction-associated fatty liver disease diagnoses and cardiovascular diseases: From epidemiology to drug approaches. Eur J Clin Invest 2021; 51(7):e13519.

7. Shao C, Wang J, Tian J, et al. Coronary artery disease: from mechanism to clinical practice. Adv Exp Med Biol 2020;1177:1–36.

8. Stefan N, Häring HU, Cusi K. Non-alcoholic fatty liver disease: causes, diagnosis, cardiometabolic consequences, and treatment strategies. Lancet Diabetes Endocrinol 2019;7(4):313–24.

9. Mantovani A, Csermely A, Petracca G, et al. Non-alcoholic fatty liver disease and risk of fatal and non-fatal cardiovascular events: an updated systematic review and meta-analysis. The Lancet Gastroenterology & Hepatology 2021;6(11): 903–13.

10. Simon TG, Roelstraete B, Hagström H, et al. Non-alcoholic fatty liver disease and incident major adverse cardiovascular events: results from a nationwide histology cohort. Gut 2022;71(9):1867–75.

11. Mantovani A, Csermely A, Tilg H, et al. Comparative effects of non-alcoholic fatty liver disease and metabolic dysfunction-associated fatty liver disease on risk of incident cardiovascular events: a meta-analysis of about 13 million individuals. Gut 2022.

12. Bedogni G, Bellentani S, Miglioli L, et al. The Fatty Liver Index: a simple and accurate predictor of hepatic steatosis in the general population. BMC Gastroenterol 2006;6:33.

13. Jeong S, Kim K, Chang J, et al. Development of a simple nonalcoholic fatty liver disease scoring system indicative of metabolic risks and insulin resistance. Ann Transl Med 2020;8(21):1414.

14. Burgess S, Foley CN, Zuber V. Inferring causal relationships between risk factors and outcomes from genome-wide association study data. Annu Rev Genomics Hum Genet 2018;19:303–27.

15. Dongiovanni P, Petta S, Maglio C, et al. Transmembrane 6 superfamily member 2 gene variant disentangles nonalcoholic steatohepatitis from cardiovascular disease. Hepatology 2015;61(2):506–14.

16. Simons N, Isaacs A, Koek GH, et al. PNPLA3, TM6SF2, and MBOAT7 genotypes and coronary artery disease. Gastroenterology 2017;152(4):912–3.

17. Romeo S, Kozlitina J, Xing C, et al. Genetic variation in PNPLA3 confers susceptibility to nonalcoholic fatty liver disease. Nat Genet 2008;40(12):1461–5.

18. Pirazzi C, Adiels M, Burza MA, et al. Patatin-like phospholipase domain-containing 3 (PNPLA3) I148M (rs738409) affects hepatic VLDL secretion in humans and in vitro. J Hepatol 2012;57(6):1276–82.

19. Speliotes EK, Yerges-Armstrong LM, Wu J, et al. Genome-wide association analysis identifies variants associated with nonalcoholic fatty liver disease that have distinct effects on metabolic traits. PLoS Genet 2011;7(3):e1001324.

20. Santoro N, Caprio S, Pierpont B, et al. Hepatic de novo lipogenesis in obese youth is modulated by a common variant in the GCKR gene. J Clin Endocrinol Metab 2015;100(8):E1125–32.

21. Simons P, Simons N, Stehouwer CDA, et al. Association of common gene variants in glucokinase regulatory protein with cardiorenal disease: A systematic review and meta-analysis. PLoS One 2018;13(10):e0206174.

22. Simons P, Valkenburg O, Stehouwer CDA, et al. Association between de novo lipogenesis susceptibility genes and coronary artery disease. Nutrition, metabolism, and cardiovascular diseases. Nutr Metab Cardiovasc Dis 2022;32(12):2883–9.

23. Brouwers M, Simons N, Stehouwer CDA, et al. Relationship between nonalcoholic fatty liver disease susceptibility genes and coronary artery disease. Hepatology Communications 2019;3(4):587–96.

24. Lauridsen BK, Stender S, Kristensen TS, et al. Liver fat content, non-alcoholic fatty liver disease, and ischaemic heart disease: mendelian randomization and meta-analysis of 279 013 individuals. Eur Heart J 2018;39(5):385–93.

25. Adiels M, Taskinen MR, Packard C, et al. Overproduction of large VLDL particles is driven by increased liver fat content in man. Diabetologia 2006;49(4):755–65.

26. Vujkovic M, Ramdas S, Lorenz KM, et al. A multiancestry genome-wide association study of unexplained chronic ALT elevation as a proxy for nonalcoholic fatty liver disease with histological and radiological validation. Nat Genet 2022;54(6):761–71.

27. Ren Z, Simons P, Wesselius A, et al. Relationship between NAFLD and coronary artery disease: a Mendelian randomization study. Hepatology 2023;77(1):230–8.

28. Promrat K, Kleiner DE, Niemeier HM, et al. Randomized controlled trial testing the effects of weight loss on nonalcoholic steatohepatitis. Hepatology 2010;51(1):121–9.

29. Li G, Zhang P, Wang J, et al. Cardiovascular mortality, all-cause mortality, and diabetes incidence after lifestyle intervention for people with impaired glucose tolerance in the Da Qing Diabetes Prevention Study: a 23-year follow-up study. Lancet Diabetes Endocrinol 2014;2(6):474–80.

30. Wing RR, Bolin P, Brancati FL, et al. Cardiovascular effects of intensive lifestyle intervention in type 2 diabetes. N Engl J Med 2013;369(2):145–54.

31. Gregg EW, Jakicic JM, Blackburn G, et al. Association of the magnitude of weight loss and changes in physical fitness with long-term cardiovascular disease outcomes in overweight or obese people with type 2 diabetes: a post-hoc analysis of the Look AHEAD randomised clinical trial. Lancet Diabetes Endocrinol 2016;4(11):913–21.

32. Mummadi RR, Kasturi KS, Chennareddygari S, et al. Effect of bariatric surgery on nonalcoholic fatty liver disease: systematic review and meta-analysis. Clin Gastroenterol Hepatol 2008;6(12):1396–402.

33. Carlsson LMS, Sjöholm K, Jacobson P, et al. Life expectancy after bariatric surgery in the swedish obese subjects study. N Engl J Med 2020;383(16):1535–43.

34. Armstrong MJ, Gaunt P, Aithal GP, et al. Liraglutide safety and efficacy in patients with non-alcoholic steatohepatitis (LEAN): a multicentre, double-blind, randomised, placebo-controlled phase 2 study. Lancet (London, England) 2016;387(10019):679–90.

35. Newsome PN, Buchholtz K, Cusi K, et al. A Placebo-Controlled Trial of Subcutaneous Semaglutide in Nonalcoholic Steatohepatitis. N Engl J Med 2021;384(12):1113–24.

36. Cusi K, Orsak B, Bril F, et al. Long-Term pioglitazone treatment for patients with nonalcoholic steatohepatitis and prediabetes or type 2 diabetes mellitus: a randomized trial. Ann Intern Med 2016;165(5):305–15.

37. Marso SP, Daniels GH, Brown-Frandsen K, et al. Liraglutide and cardiovascular outcomes in type 2 diabetes. N Engl J Med 2016;375(4):311–22.
38. Marso SP, Bain SC, Consoli A, et al. Semaglutide and cardiovascular outcomes in patients with type 2 diabetes. N Engl J Med 2016;375(19):1834–44.
39. Kernan WN, Viscoli CM, Furie KL, et al. Pioglitazone after ischemic stroke or transient ischemic attack. N Engl J Med 2016;374(14):1321–31.
40. Dormandy JA, Charbonnel B, Eckland DJ, et al. Secondary prevention of macrovascular events in patients with type 2 diabetes in the PROactive Study (PROspective pioglitAzone Clinical Trial In macroVascular Events): a randomised controlled trial. Lancet (London, England) 2005;366(9493):1279–89.
41. van Dalem J, Driessen JHM, Burden AM, et al. Thiazolidinediones and glucagon-like peptide-1 receptor agonists and the risk of nonalcoholic fatty liver disease: a cohort study. Hepatology 2021;74(5):2467–77.
42. EASL-EASD-EASO. EASL-EASD-EASO Clinical Practice Guidelines for the management of non-alcoholic fatty liver disease. J Hepatol 2016;64(6):1388–402.
43. Younossi ZM, Corey KE, Lim JK. AGA clinical practice update on lifestyle modification using diet and exercise to achieve weight loss in the management of nonalcoholic fatty liver disease: expert review. Gastroenterology 2021;160(3): 912–8.
44. Cusi K, Isaacs S, Barb D, et al. American association of clinical endocrinology clinical practice guideline for the diagnosis and management of nonalcoholic fatty liver disease in primary care and endocrinology clinical settings: co-sponsored by the american association for the study of liver diseases (AASLD). Endocr Pract 2022;28(5):528–62.
45. Arnett DK, Blumenthal RS, Albert MA, et al. 2019 ACC/AHA guideline on the primary prevention of cardiovascular disease: a report of the american college of cardiology/american heart association task force on clinical practice guidelines. Circulation 2019;140(11):e596–646.
46. Luijten J, van Greevenbroek MMJ, Schaper NC, et al. Incidence of cardiovascular disease in familial combined hyperlipidemia: A 15-year follow-up study. Atherosclerosis 2019;280:1–6.
47. Ahmad OS, Morris JA, Mujammami M, et al. A Mendelian randomization study of the effect of type-2 diabetes on coronary heart disease. Nat Commun 2015;6: 7060.
48. Shah AD, Langenberg C, Rapsomaniki E, et al. Type 2 diabetes and incidence of cardiovascular diseases: a cohort study in 1·9 million people. Lancet Diabetes Endocrinol 2015;3(2):105–13.
49. Visseren FLJ, Mach F, Smulders YM, et al. 2021 ESC Guidelines on cardiovascular disease prevention in clinical practice. Eur Heart J 2021;42(34):3227–337.
50. Athyros VG, Tziomalos K, Gossios TD, et al. Safety and efficacy of long-term statin treatment for cardiovascular events in patients with coronary heart disease and abnormal liver tests in the Greek Atorvastatin and Coronary Heart Disease Evaluation (GREACE) Study: a post-hoc analysis. Lancet (London, England) 2010;376(9756):1916–22.
51. Bays H, Cohen DE, Chalasani N, et al. An assessment by the statin liver safety task force: 2014 update. Journal of Clinical Lipidology 2014;8(3 Suppl):S47–57.
52. Ekstedt M, Hagström H, Nasr P, et al. Fibrosis stage is the strongest predictor for disease-specific mortality in NAFLD after up to 33 years of follow-up. Hepatology 2015;61(5):1547–54.

Metabolic-Associated Fatty Liver Disease and Diabetes
A Double Whammy

Nitin Kapoor, MD(Medicine), DM(Endocrinology), PhD(University of Melbourne)[a,b],
Sanjay Kalra, MD(Medicine), DM(Endocrinology)[c,d],*

KEYWORDS

- Metabolic-associated fatty liver disease • Metabolic syndrome • Fatty liver
- Type 2 diabetes mellitus • Obesity

KEY POINTS

- Metabolic-associated fatty liver disease (MAFLD) and type 2 diabetes mellitus frequently tend to coexist, potentiating adverse outcomes and individual progression of both disorders.
- MAFLD is the most common cause of chronic liver disease in children and adolescents but can be effectively prevented with lifestyle modifications.
- Several biomarkers like SteatoTest/fatty liver index can be used in clinical practice to suspect MAFLD even in resource-limited settings.
- In addition to lifestyle modifications, pharmacologic interventions including certain antidiabetic agents, antihyperlipidaemic drugs, and some novel targeted agents in addition to bariatric procedures have been successful in the management of MAFLD.

INTRODUCTION

Fatty liver (FL) disease is a widely prevalent disorder first described in 1980s,[1] but more recently, the prevalence has increased several fold affecting almost a quarter of the global population. Initially referred to as nonalcoholic FL disease (NAFLD) over the years, with a better understanding of the disease process, the nomenclature has been changed and is more appropriately referred to as metabolic (dysfunction)-associated FL disease (MAFLD).[2] This is more relevant when investigated in the presence of

Both authors declare no conflict of interest or funding disclosures for this article.
a Department of Endocrinology, Diabetes and Metabolism, Christian Medical College, Vellore, TN 632004, India; b Non communicable disease unit, Baker Heart and Diabetes Institute, Melbourne, VIC 3004, Australia; c Department of Endocrinology, Bharti Hospital, Endocrine Society of India (ESI), Bharti Hospital & B.R.I.D.E, Karnal, India; d University Center for Research & Development, Chandigarh University, South Asian Federation of Endocrine Societies (SAFES), India
* Corresponding author. Bharti Hospital, Endocrine Society of India (ESI), Bharti Hospital & B.R. I.D.E, Karnal, Haryana, India-132001.
E-mail address: brideknl@gmail.com

diabetes mellitus. Although there are subtle differences between the two diagnoses, MAFLD seems to be a more appropriate term encompassing its heterogeneous pathogenesis and appropriate stratification of patients from a management standpoint.[3]

The two most significant differences in the diagnostic criteria between MAFLD and NAFLD are that MAFLD diagnosis does not require exclusion of patients with alcohol intake or other chronic liver disorders such as viral hepatitis. Furthermore, the presence of a metabolic abnormality (eg, type 2 diabetes mellitus [T2DM]) is necessary for diagnosis of MAFLD.[4] The diagnostic criteria for MAFLD are summarized in **Table 1** and are considered as the hepatic manifestation of metabolic syndrome.[5]

MAFLD encompasses a disease spectrum from hepatic steatosis to hepatitis, fibrosis, cirrhosis, and at times even malignancy (**Fig. 1**).[5]

Hepatic steatosis is an abnormal liver fat that exceeds 5% of the total liver weight or 5% of hepatocytes are laden with fat. Although ideal to diagnose this stage on histopathology, both imaging techniques and noninvasive biological scores are able to predict this with fair amount of accuracy. Nonalcoholic steatohepatitis (NASH) is defined by the histological presence of three components in the liver including steatosis, hepatocyte ballooning, and hepatocellular inflammation. Similarly, even fibrosis ideally requires histopathological examination but can be well predicted by using clinical-bio markers and/or imaging techniques using age-appropriate cutoffs. Cirrhosis is characterized by diffuse nodular regeneration surrounded by dense fibrotic septa associated with pronounced distortion of hepatic vascular architecture. Cirrhosis remains asymptomatic until decompensation occurs due to portal hypertension or is detected during routine master health check. Furthermore, hepatocellular carcinoma could occur after cirrhosis or even bypassing the stage of cirrhosis directly after the stage of NASH.

PROBLEM STATEMENT OF METABOLIC-ASSOCIATED FATTY LIVER DISEASE AND DIABETES

MAFLD is the most common liver disease globally. Its prevalence has been rapidly increasing in parallel to the epidemics of diabetes and obesity. A meta-analysis by Younossi and colleagues,[6] on the prevalence of NAFLD in patients with T2DM, suggested the global prevalence to be about 55%, of whom 37.3% had NASH and approximately 4.8% had advanced fibrosis. The investigators in yet another study projected that about 18.2 million people in United States had both T2DM and MAFLD.[7] Over the next two decades, it is estimated that NASH with T2DM would account for 1.37 million cardiovascular deaths and 81,200 liver-related deaths. Similar estimates have been made from other countries as well.[8] In a recently published cohort study, it was shown that individuals with MAFLD had a 14% higher risk of cardiovascular mortality than non-MAFLD individuals.[9]

A meta-analysis on global prevalence by Lim and colleagues[10] reported a pooled prevalence of MAFLD in 39.2%, with the highest prevalence in Europe and Asia followed by North America. The MAFLD prevalence accounted for 81.59% of all individuals having NAFLD. MAFLD was found to be significantly associated with male sex,

Table 1 Diagnostic criteria for metabolic-associated fatty liver disease	
1	Evidence of hepatic steatosis based on clinical/laboratory parameters and/or liver histology
2	Presence of a metabolic risk condition, for example, overweight/obesity and/or type 2 diabetes mellitus and/or any of the components of metabolic syndrome

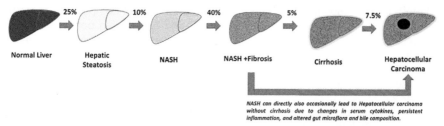

Fig. 1. The disease spectrum of metabolic-associated fatty liver disease (MAFLD). NASH, nonalcoholic steatohepatitis.

higher body mass index (BMI), presence of hypertension, diabetes, dyslipidemia, transaminitis, and greater fibrosis score compared with patients with NAFLD.[10]

LIVER PANCREAS CROSS TALK

There is a significant contribution of liver dysfunction in the development of T2DM. Although these mechanisms are not fully understood, hepatic fat accumulation leads to alterations in energy metabolism and inflammatory signals that contribute to insulin resistance. Moreover, chronic hyperinsulinemia as seen in patients with T2DM also leads to hepatic fat accretion. Lipotoxins, mitochondrial dysfunction, cytokines, and adipocytokines have been proposed to play a major role in the pathogenesis of both MAFLD and T2DM. Based on a recent review by Byrne and colleagues,[11] a diagrammatic representation of the risk of developing diabetes and MAFLD in the presence of each other is depicted in **Fig. 2**. A higher baseline FL index has been shown to be an independent predictor of developing new onset diabetes during a 10 year follow-up.

METABOLIC SYNDROME AND METABOLIC-ASSOCIATED FATTY LIVER DISEASE

Individual studies have shown that MAFLD has been associated with obesity, dyslipidemia, hypertension, and diabetes all of which have been individually associated with metabolic syndrome (MetS), such that it has been considered the hepatic manifestation of the MetS.[12] There is growing evidence that this relationship between MAFLD

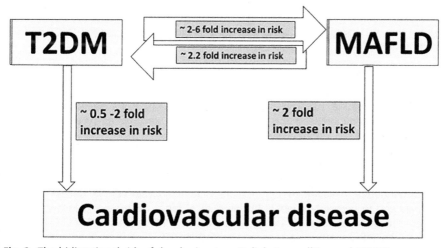

Fig. 2. The bidirectional risk of developing type 2 diabetes mellitus and MAFLD.

and MetS is bidirectional. MAFLD can predispose to different components of MetS, which can in turn exacerbate MAFLD. Although the relationship between MAFLD and MetS is considered bidirectional, recently there has been much interest in genotype/phenotype relationships where there is a disconnect between the liver disease and MetS features. This has been shown with genotypes such as patatin-like phospholipase domain-containing protein-3 (I148M) and transmembrane 6 superfamily member 2 protein (E167K).[13]

Evaluation of Metabolic (Dysfunction)-Associated Fatty Liver Disease in Presence of Diabetes

The following biochemical and radiological tools help to make a diagnosis of MAFLD. These investigations are used not only for diagnosis but also to follow-up and determine the severity in affected patients.

Serum Biomarkers

Even though at present there is no single ideal biomarker that can be used to diagnose MAFLD, there are certain noninvasive models that are proposed to help better prediction of steatosis. The most common biochemical parameter that raises a suspicion of underlying hepatic steatosis is the presence of elevated alanine aminotransferase. In a recent article by Zeng and colleagues,[14] several biomarkers that predict MAFLD have been described. Some of these are for clinical use, and others used as research tools have been described. These have been categorized as apoptosis biomarkers, fibrosis biomarkers, inflammatory biomarkers, adipokines and hepatokines, genomics, epigenomics, transcriptomics, and proteomics. Some clinically useful biomarkers have been described below.

SteatoTest: This is a logistic regression model comprising 12 clinical and biochemical parameters including age, sex, BMI, alanine aminotransferase, alpha-2 macroglobulin, apolipoprotein A1, haptoglobin, total bilirubin, gamma-glutamyl transferase, cholesterol, serum triglycerides, and blood glucose. In a study by Poynard and colleagues,[15] the SteatoTest had a sensitivity and specificity of 90% among 884 NAFLD subjects. The advantage of this tool is that it is noninvasive and uses easily available parameters in these patients.

Fatty liver index: This is based on a more simplified validated algorithm-based index derived from minimal indices including BMI, waist circumference, serum triglyceride levels, and gamma-glutamyl transferase. This index varies from 0 to 100 and a value of more than 60 is suggestive of FL disease. This has also been previously compared with the SteatoTest.

Imaging Modalities

Ultrasonography: This is a widely used technique for screening individuals who are suspected to have MAFLD. The underlying principle is that in the presence of excessive fat, there is an increased echogenicity of the liver, which in turn makes it appear brighter as compared with the renal cortex.[16]

Several studies have shown a sensitivity varying from 91% to 100%, which makes ultrasound a good screening tool.[17–19] It is preferred because it is noninvasive, relatively less expensive, and widely available. The major limiting factors include its operator dependence, inability to differentiate diffuse fibrosis versus diffuse hepatic steatosis and to precisely quantify the amount of fat at baseline and follow-up.[20] It is often difficult to interpret in obesity, which is often the case with MAFLD.[21]

A more objective method on sonography to detect FL is a hepato-renal ratio (HRR). This is based on the principle that in normal circumstances, the liver and kidney have a similar echogenicity. In the presence of FL, the liver will appear brighter than the renal parenchyma. HRR has shown to have 100% sensitivity and 91% specificity for the diagnosis of hepatic steatosis.[22]

Vibration controlled transient elastography (VCTE)/fibroscan: Transient elastography is a noninvasive technique to measure the hepatic tissue elasticity and thereby predict the degree of fibrosis (liver stiffness). Although the liver stiffness was initially proposed as a reliable tool to identify fibrosis and cirrhosis in patients with hepatitis C, now data are also evident for its use in MAFLD.[23] The only major limiting factor in its use in patients with MAFLD is the usually high BMI associated in these patients which may underestimate the disease burden due to the attenuation of the ultrasound waves. Controlled attenuation parameter is a similar tool based on liver stiffness measurement that has been developed to use with a fibroscan. Its value may range from 100 to 400 decibels per meter (Db/M). A cutoff value more than 283 Db/M has shown to have a sensitivity of 76% and a specificity of 79% to detect steatosis.[24] The use of ultrasound elastography is a promising tool in most types of liver disease as in MAFLD; however, it has its own limitations especially in individuals with obesity, which may lead to underdiagnosis and thereby underestimation of primary MAFLD rates.

Computed tomography scan: Computed tomography (CT) scan provides a vivid assessment of the entire liver making it possible for even small amounts of focal infiltrations to be picked up in addition to diffuse involvement. Unlike the ultrasound, the CT scan measures the attenuation difference in contrast to spleen and not the kidney in terms of Hounsfield units.[25] This is best visualized in the non-contrast images where hepatic fat appears as hypodense areas on the liver. It has been shown to have a sensitivity of 73% to 100% and a specificity of 95% to 100% to detect moderate to severe steatosis.[26] However, despite a good pick-up rate, its role in practice for diagnosis of FL is limited by its cost and radiation exposure both of which make it difficult to use it even during follow-up.

Magnetic resonance imaging scan: Several studies have demonstrated that two-dimensional magnetic resonance (MR) elastography may be a promising biomarker in the noninvasive diagnosis of advanced fibrosis in MAFLD, with modest success in the diagnosis of NASH.[27] However, despite its good sensitivity and specificity, its cost and limited availability is a major limiting factor. MRE and vibration-controlled transient elastography have been shown to have an excellent diagnostic performance for assessing hepatic fibrosis in patients with morbid obesity.[28] In a study by Chen and colleagues,[28] MRE has been shown to be technically more reliable than vibration-controlled transient elastography (VCTE).

Magnetic resonance spectroscopy: This is another tool that has been validated to assess the hepatic fat content in individuals with MetS. Although magnetic resonance spectroscopy (MRS) was initially designed for cranial imaging, the proton-based 1H MRS is currently being used in the research setting to reliably asses the hepatic fat content.[29]

Liver biopsy: Liver biopsy remains the gold standard for the diagnosis and staging of NASH and to capture the degree of fibrosis due to the lack of many precise noninvasive measures to do that. NASH is characterized by ballooning of hepatocytes and lobular inflammation with or without perisinusoidal fibrosis in the background of steatosis. Although liver biopsy is not warranted in all patients with NASH due to its cost, invasive nature, and associated risks, the physician's discretion is required to balance between the risks and benefits in any given patient.[30] Liver biopsy may also rule out other associated causes (sero-negative autoimmune hepatitis, chronic hepatitis B or C virus infection, Wilson disease, drug-induced liver injury, and alpha-1-antitrypsin deficiency) of chronic liver disease in MAFLD.

Management of Metabolic-Associated Fatty Liver Disease with Type 2 Diabetes Mellitus

Lifestyle interventions

Lifestyle modification is the first-line of treatment of all patients with MAFLD. It often is the only intervention needed for a majority of these patients. Moreover, it needs to be continued even when other modalities of treatment are added.[31] In a study by Gomez and colleagues, where the impact of lifestyle intervention was studied prospectively in 293 patients after a year of weight loss, 25% achieved resolution of steatohepatitis, 47% had reductions in NAFLD score, and about 20% had regression in fibrosis. The maximum reduction in MAFLD-related parameters was observed in patients who had a weight loss more than 10%.[32]

The impact of dietary interventions in patients with diabetes and metabolic-associated fatty liver disease

Over the years, dietary interventions for managing noncommunicable disorders have evolved from a general disease-related advice to a patient-centric, customized dietary plan.[33] Several studies have tested which diet would work better for the management of MAFLD. A recent systematic review by Varkaneh and colleagues compared the efficacy of low carbohydrate versus low-fat interventions. The investigators concluded that the use of low-calorie diet, irrespective of fat and carbohydrate content, resulted in similar outcomes. Although both reduced body weight and liver fat content, low-fat diet was more successful in reducing the transaminase levels.[34] Similar results have also been shown with other diets including the Mediterranean diet, intermittent fasting, and other very low-calorie diets.[35–38] However, further studies that robustly evaluate the impact of these diets along with their acceptability, sustainability, and the effect on the patients' health-related quality of life are needed.[39]

EXERCISE-RELATED INTERVENTIONS FOR THE MANAGEMENT OF METABOLIC-ASSOCIATED FATTY LIVER DISEASE WITH DIABETES

Different exercise-related interventions have been tried in patients with MAFLD. Those that result in high-intensity energy expenditure and contribute to significant weight loss have been more beneficial. In a meta-analysis by Zhou and colleagues,[40] analyzing 17 studies with 1627 patients found that a combination of aerobic with resistance exercise followed by high-intensity interval training was most efficient in improving liver-related parameters. Another study by Hong and colleagues,[41] which demonstrated the beneficial effects of exercise training in patients with NAFLD, showed that the benefits were more marked in younger individuals than older patients. The key differences in the use of lifestyle interventions in patients with MAFLD with diabetes as compared with those without diabetes is that the intensity of interventions required for patients with MAFLD would often be twice as intense (5% weight loss for patients with diabetes versus 10% weight loss for MAFLD).

PHARMACOTHERAPY FOR THE MANAGEMENT OF METABOLIC-ASSOCIATED FATTY LIVER DISEASE IN PATIENTS WITH TYPE 2 DIABETES MELLITUS

The Utility of Antidiabetic Agents in the Management of Metabolic-Associated Fatty Liver Disease

A brief summary on the current evidence on the utility of commonly used management strategies of managing MAFLD in patients with diabetes mellitus are summarized in **Table 2.**

Table 2
Summary of the current evidence of different management strategies commonly used in patients with diabetes to address metabolic-associated fatty liver disease

Management Strategy	Current Evidence	Recommendation
Lifestyle interventions		
Dietary modifications	• Low-calorie diet irrespective of the macronutrient proportions that results in more than 10% weight loss is helpful in improving MAFLD-related parameters in patients with diabetes	• More studies needed to evaluate the impact of these diets along with their acceptability, sustainability, and the effect on health-related quality of life.
Exercise interventions	• Helpful in patients with MAFLD when coupled with a hypocaloric diet especially in younger adults; follow-up studies of 24 months.	• Long-term follow-up is needed to derive more meaningful conclusions.
Pharmacotherapy		
Pioglitazone	• Pioglitazone is recommended for treatment of MAFLD when there is evidence of nonalcoholic steatohepatitis (NASH) especially in the presence of T2DM.	• Side effects are problems including water retention, and increased risk of fragility fracture. Contraindications: Significant stages of congestive cardiac failure and wet maculopathy
Metformin (also recommended in non-MAFLD)	• Improves insulin resistance, hepatic enzymes, and body weight	• Not primarily recommended for patients with NASH though considered in treatment of diabetes with MAFLD and NASH
Dipeptidyl peptidase-IV (DPP-IV) inhibitors	• No significant improvement in MAFLD-related parameters • Not recommended to use in patients for management of MAFLD • No improvement in liver histology	• Not primarily recommended for patients with NASH though considered in treatment of diabetes with MAFLD and NASH
Glucagon-like peptide-1 analogs	• Improvement in MAFLD-related parameters likely due to associated weight loss.	• Recommended for the management of NASH, but to also explain the patient about the gastrointestinal(GI) side effects and high cost

(continued on next page)

Table 2
(continued)

Management Strategy	Current Evidence	Recommendation
Sodium–glucose cotransporter-2 (SGLT2) inhibitors	• Significant reduction in transaminitis and fibrosis-4 score(FIB-4) index	• Very useful in type 2 diabetes management • Need for long-term studies to prove its sustained benefit.
Insulin	• No evidence to support improvement in MAFLD-related parameters	• Used for control of diabetes
Alpha-glucosidase inhibitors	• No evidence to support improvement in MAFLD-related parameters	• Can be used for the management of diabetes as needed
Sulphonylureas	• No evidence to support improvement in MAFLD-related parameters	• To be used with caution in patients with liver disease as most of these drugs are metabolized in the liver

Pioglitazone

The peroxisome proliferator-activated receptors gamma agonists are insulin sensitizers used in the management of T2DM. Pioglitazone is the only drug in this class of thiazolidinediones widely available. A recently published systematic review and meta-analysis by Kovalic and colleagues, summarizing 40 randomized clinical trials, reported that the relative risk of 45 mg pioglitazone in reducing a two-point improvement in NAFLD activity score was 3.29 (95% CI 1.74–6,22) and 2.65 (95% CI 1.36–5.12) for NASH resolution without worsening fibrosis. Currently, pioglitazone is recommended for treatment of MAFLD when there is evidence of NASH especially in the presence of T2DM.[42] However, its known adverse effects of water retention, limited use in patients with significant congestive cardiac failure and increased risk of osteoporosis have to be kept in mind before its rampant use.

Metformin

Metformin, a biguanide is one of the most widely prescribed drugs for the management of T2DM. Given its euglycemic nature, associated weight loss, efficient glycemic control, lower cost, and a beta cell sparing action makes it one of the most ideal antidiabetic agents available today. However, in the setting of MAFLD, it has only shown to improve liver function, insulin sensitivity, and body weight. There has been no histological improvement in patients with NASH and T2DM and hence not recommended for specifically treating MAFLD.[42]

Dipeptidyl Peptidase-IV Inhibitors

Although incretin physiology has been known for several years, its pharmacologic manipulation has been an area of great research in the past few decades. The endogenously secreted incretin hormones are degraded by the enzyme dipeptidyl peptidase-IV (DPP-IV), and thereby by inhibiting this enzyme, the physiological action of the endogenously produced glucagon-like peptide-1 (GLP-1) can be enhanced. Although DPP-IVi has several advantages for use in patients with T2DM including weight neutrality, less incidence of hypoglycemia, and low cost, they have not been found to be very beneficial in patients with MAFLD. In a recently published meta-analysis including 40 randomized clinical trials, it was found that DDP-IVi did not show significant improvements in MAFLD-related parameters in patients with T2DM and hence not recommended for use in this setting.[43]

Glucagon-like peptide-1 analogs

GLP-1 analogs are currently the most effective noninsulin antidiabetic agents that in addition to control blood glucose, also help attaining significant weight loss.[44,45] They work by enhancing the incretin physiology and have been studied extensively for their utility in patients with MAFLD. Significant weight reduction caused by GLP-1 analogs is said to be one of the main reasons for improvements in MAFLD. A recent meta-analysis composing of 40 randomized clinical trials showed a significant reduction in liver enzymes and FIB-4 index unlike DPP-IVi.[43]

As per the recent AACE guidelines, these drugs are recommended for the management of NASH, moreover they also provide good glycemic control, modest weight loss, and other cardiometabolic benefits. However, cost is still a limiting factor especially in the developing world.[46] Moreover, gastrointestinal side effects along with other side effects may result in a discontinuation rate of about 5 to 10% during the course of treatment.[42]

Sodium–Glucose Cotransporter-2 Inhibitors

SGLT-2is are antidiabetic agents that in addition to reduction in glucose provide cardio-renal protection and also promote mild weight loss in a non-islet cell-dependent manner.[47] A recent meta-analysis comparing the efficacy of newer antidiabetic agents in improvement of MAFLD has shown remarkable reduction in transaminitis and FIB-4 index with the use of sodium–glucose cotransporter-2 inhibitors. Although preliminary studies seem promising, long-term data are warranted to prove their sustained efficacy in MAFLD despite only a modest weight loss.[43]

Summarizing, SGLT2-inhibitors are likely to control diabetes and also benefit MAFLD.

THE UTILITY OF OTHER DRUGS (NOT ANTIDIABETIC AGENTS) IN THE MANAGEMENT OF METABOLIC-ASSOCIATED FATTY LIVER DISEASE

Although management of MAFLD in patients with diabetes requires the optimal choice of antidiabetic agents, certain other agents have also been tried. **Table 3** summaries the current evidence for the utility of these drugs in clinical practice to manage MAFLD in the presence of diabetes.[42]

BARIATRIC SURGERY AND INTRAGASTRIC PROCEDURES

Currently, bariatric procedures are the most effective methods to reduce weight in patients with severe obesity. The drastic weight reduction after these procedures helps in remission of several metabolic disorders such as, T2DM dyslipidemia, obstructive sleep apnea, and even MAFLD.

The two common bariatric surgery procedures include the Roux-en-Y gastric bypass and sleeve gastrectomy (SG). However, these are indicated for specific obesity status and not for MAFLD.[51]

Similarly, less invasive endoscopic bariatric procedures such as intragastric balloon are increasingly performed worldwide.[52] These have fewer surgical side effects and help to attain a significant weight loss. Although long-term data on outcomes of MAFLD-related parameters for them are still not available, short-term data seem promising for patients in whom these are indicated otherwise.

MANAGEMENT OF METABOLIC-ASSOCIATED FATTY LIVER DISEASE AMONG PATIENTS WITH DIABETES IN SPECIAL SITUATIONS
Gestational Diabetes and Metabolic-Associated Fatty Liver Disease

Gestational diabetes has a significant impact on both the mother and the fetus. The presence of MAFLD is associated with a further increase in the risk of developing pregnancy-induced hypertension, postpartum hemorrhage, and premature delivery due to the underlying insulin resistance parameters. In a study by Lee and colleagues,[53] it was found that about one in five women in pregnancy had MAFLD and its presence was found to be an independent risk factor for the presence of gestational diabetes. Moreover, in another study by Mosca and colleagues,[54] it was shown that fetus exposed to MAFLD in the mother had a greater risk of developing obesity and MAFLD in early childhood.

Type 1 Diabetes and Metabolic-Associated Fatty Liver Disease

Although MAFLD is largely considered as a hepatic manifestation of MetS, it has also been reported in patients with type 1 diabetes mellitus (T1DM).[55–57] About a third of patients with T1DM have MAFLD, but the prevalence varies largely depending on

Table 3
Summary of the current evidence of nondiabetic agents in the treatment of metabolic-associated fatty liver disease

Management Strategy	Key Points Summarizing the Current Evidence	Recommendations
Statins and other antihyperlipidemic drugs	• Improves steatosis grade and NAFLD activity score[48]	• Should be considered in all patients except those with transaminitis (>3 times the upper limit of normal) • More evidence is needed for other antihyperlipidemic drugs such as fenofibrate and pro-protein convertase subtilisin/kexin type 9 inhibitors
Vitamin E/alpha-tocopherol	• Associated with worsening of insulin resistance[49]	• Not recommended in patients with diabetes[46]
Orlistat	• Conflicting results in favor and against its use[50]	• Encouraging data from basic science and animal experiments suggest further testing in long-term clinical trials.
Obeticholic acid	• Bile acid mimic shows encouraging results in short-term studies • Could be a potential treatment option in future for patients with MAFLD, considering that it reduces fatty liver and liver fibrosis	• No role in control of DM
Aldafermin (FGF-19 analog)	• Activates farnesoid X receptor (FXR) receptors and simulates actions like fibroblast growth factor 19 (FGF19)	• Short-term initial studies look promising for its future use (for MAFLD?)

the age and BMI of the study cohort.[58,59] Although increasing insulin resistance in relatively older patients with T1DM is described as an important risk factor for the development of MAFLD, even oxidative stress, poor glycemic control, genetic predisposition, and exogenous insulin administration also play a role. An entity called glycogenic hepatopathy (liver dysfunction in poorly controlled T1DM) is a close differential diagnosis in such patients. The evaluation and management of MAFLD in patients with T1DM is similar to those with T2DM.[60]

OUTCOMES OF METABOLIC-ASSOCIATED FATTY LIVER DISEASE IN PATIENTS WITH DIABETES AS COMPARED WITH THOSE WITHOUT DIABETES

Multiple studies have shown that the prevalence of MAFLD is two to three-fold more common in patients with diabetes as compared with those without diabetes. In a recent study by Ajmera and colleagues,[61] about 65% of individuals were found to be affected using the MRI-based assessment of liver fat. Furthermore, several studies have demonstrated that the MAFLD-associated severity, morbidity, progression, and liver-related mortality are much higher in patients with diabetes.[61–63]

Lean Metabolic-Associated Fatty Liver Disease and Diabetes

Although MAFLD is conventionally described in people with obesity, it may less often also be associated in individuals with an apparently lean phenotype.[64] This is especially peculiar in the south Asian phenotype, wherein individuals may have high body fat despite a normal BMI.[65] The body fat percentage in these individuals is significantly high and is often deposited in ectopic sites such as the liver, muscle, heart, omentum, and kidney.[66] The response to lifestyle interventions in such individuals is often more difficult.[67,68]

SUMMARY

MAFLD is a major public health issue especially in patients with diabetes. It is essential to screen and evaluate patients with diabetes, even in cost-restrained settings using simple screening tools such as ultrasound or fibroscan and biomarkers. The more recently available antidiabetic agents including GLP-1 analogs and SGLT-2is have been shown to be effective in both diabetes and MAFLD. Beyond antidiabetic agents, newer drugs such as FGF-19 analogs and bariatric/endoscopic procedures for obesity have also been shown effective in reduction of MAFLD-related parameters in DM. Long-term studies are needed to determine their efficacy and safety for routine clinical use.

CLINICS CARE POINTS

- The prevalence of metabolic-associated fatty liver disease (MAFLD) is approximately 55% in patients with type 2 diabetes mellitus and represents a spectrum of disorders ranging from hepatic steatosis to hepatitis, fibrosis, cirrhosis, and hepatocellular carcinoma.

- All patients with diabetes should be screened for MAFLD and vice versa. Several serum biomarkers and radiological modalities have been suggested for screening, depending on the clinical setting.

- Antidiabetic agents such as pioglitazone, glucagon-like peptide-1 analogs, and sodium–glucose cotransporter-2 inhibitors have shown significant improvement in MAFLD-related parameters in patients with diabetes. Newer drugs and endoscopic/bariatric procedures also have shown to be helpful in short-term studies.

REFERENCES

1. Ludwig J, Viggiano TR, McGill DB, et al. Nonalcoholic steatohepatitis: Mayo Clinic experiences with a hitherto unnamed disease. Mayo Clin Proc 1980; 55(7):434–8.
2. Eslam M, Sanyal AJ, George J. MAFLD: a consensus-driven proposed nomenclature for metabolic-associated fatty liver disease. Gastroenterology 2020;158(7): 1999–2014.e1991.
3. Lin S, Huang J, Wang M, et al. Comparison of MAFLD and NAFLD diagnostic criteria in real world. Liver Int 2020;40(9):2082–9.
4. Eslam M, Newsome PN, Sarin SK, et al. A new definition for metabolic dysfunction-associated fatty liver disease: an international expert consensus statement. J Hepatol 2020;73(1):202–9.
5. Binet Q, Loumaye A, Preumont V, et al. Non-invasive screening, staging and management of metabolic dysfunction-associated fatty liver disease (MAFLD) in type 2 diabetes mellitus patients: what do we know so far. Acta Gastroenterol Belg 2022;85(2):346–57.
6. Younossi ZM, Golabi P, de Avila L, et al. The global epidemiology of NAFLD and NASH in patients with type 2 diabetes: a systematic review and meta-analysis. J Hepatol 2019;71(4):793–801.
7. Younossi ZM, Tampi RP, Racila A, et al. Economic and clinical burden of nonalcoholic steatohepatitis in patients with type 2 diabetes in the U.S. Diabetes Care 2020;43(2):283–9.
8. Vandekerckhove P, Van Damme B, Annemans L. How will the welfare state cope with welfare diseases such as NASH? Acta Gastroenterol Belg 2019;82(4):548–9.
9. Yoo TK, Lee MY, Kim SH, et al. Comparison of cardiovascular mortality between MAFLD and NAFLD: a cohort study. Nutr Metab Cardiovasc Dis 2023;00024–8.
10. Lim GEH, Tang A, Ng CH, et al. An observational data meta-analysis on the differences in prevalence and risk factors between MAFLD vs NAFLD. Clin Gastroenterol Hepatol 2021;00024–8.
11. Byrne CD. Banting memorial lecture 2022: 'type 2 diabetes and nonalcoholic fatty liver disease: partners in crime'. Diabet Med 2022;39(10):e14912.
12. Godoy-Matos AF, Silva Júnior WS, Valerio CM. NAFLD as a continuum: from obesity to metabolic syndrome and diabetes. Diabetol Metab Syndrome 2020; 12:60.
13. Wainwright P, Byrne CD. Bidirectional relationships and disconnects between NAFLD and features of the metabolic syndrome. Int J Mol Sci 2016;17(3):367.
14. Zeng Y, He H, An Z. Advance of serum biomarkers and combined diagnostic panels in nonalcoholic fatty liver disease. Dis Markers 2022;2022:1254014.
15. Poynard T, Peta V, Deckmyn O, et al. Performance of liver biomarkers, in patients at risk of nonalcoholic steato-hepatitis, according to presence of type-2 diabetes. Eur J Gastroenterol Hepatol 2020;32(8):998–1007.
16. Quinn SF, Gosink BB. Characteristic sonographic signs of hepatic fatty infiltration. AJR Am J Roentgenol 1985;145(4):753–5.
17. Jimba S, Nakagami T, Takahashi M, et al. Prevalence of non-alcoholic fatty liver disease and its association with impaired glucose metabolism in Japanese adults. Diabet Med 2005;22(9):1141–5.
18. Saadeh S, Younossi ZM, Remer EM, et al. The utility of radiological imaging in nonalcoholic fatty liver disease. Gastroenterology 2002;123(3):745–50.

19. Wu J, You J, Yerian L, et al. Prevalence of liver steatosis and fibrosis and the diagnostic accuracy of ultrasound in bariatric surgery patients. Obes Surg 2012; 22(2):240–7.
20. Palmentieri B, de Sio I, La Mura V, et al. The role of bright liver echo pattern on ultrasound B-mode examination in the diagnosis of liver steatosis. Dig Liver Dis 2006;38(7):485–9.
21. Atri A, Jiwanmall SA, Nandyal MB, et al. The prevalence and predictors of non-alcoholic fatty liver disease in morbidly obese women - a cross-sectional study from Southern India. Eur Endocrinol 2020;16(2):152–5.
22. Borges VF, Diniz AL, Cotrim HP, et al. Sonographic hepatorenal ratio: a noninvasive method to diagnose nonalcoholic steatosis. J Clin Ultrasound 2013;41(1): 18–25.
23. Sandrin L, Fourquet B, Hasquenoph JM, et al. Transient elastography: a new noninvasive method for assessment of hepatic fibrosis. Ultrasound Med Biol 2003;29(12):1705–13.
24. Myers RP, Pollett A, Kirsch R, et al. Controlled Attenuation Parameter (CAP): a noninvasive method for the detection of hepatic steatosis based on transient elastography. Liver Int 2012;32(6):902–10.
25. Fierbinteanu-Braticevici C, Dina I, Petrisor A, et al. Noninvasive investigations for nonalcoholic fatty liver disease and liver fibrosis. World J Gastroenterol 2010; 16(38):4784–91.
26. Roldan-Valadez E, Favila R, Martínez-López M, et al. Imaging techniques for assessing hepatic fat content in nonalcoholic fatty liver disease. Ann Hepatol 2008; 7(3):212–20.
27. Loomba R, Sirlin CB, Ang B, et al. Ezetimibe for the treatment of nonalcoholic steatohepatitis: assessment by novel magnetic resonance imaging and magnetic resonance elastography in a randomized trial (MOZART trial). Hepatology 2015; 61(4):1239–50.
28. Chen J, Yin M, Talwalkar JA, et al. Diagnostic performance of MR elastography and vibration-controlled transient elastography in the detection of hepatic fibrosis in patients with severe to morbid obesity. Radiology 2017;283(2):418–28.
29. Makhija N, Vikram NK, Srivastava DN, et al. Role of diffusion-weighted magnetic resonance imaging in the diagnosis and grading of hepatic steatosis in patients with non-alcoholic fatty liver disease: comparison with ultrasonography and magnetic resonance spectroscopy. J Clin Exp Hepatol 2021;11(6):654–60.
30. Kleiner DE, Brunt EM, Van Natta M, et al. Design and validation of a histological scoring system for nonalcoholic fatty liver disease. Hepatology 2005;41(6): 1313–21.
31. Kapoor N, Sahay R, Kalra S, et al. Consensus on medical nutrition therapy for diabesity (CoMeND) in adults: a South Asian perspective. Diabetes Metab Syndr Obes 2021;14:1703–28.
32. Vilar-Gomez E, Martinez-Perez Y, Calzadilla-Bertot L, et al. Weight loss through lifestyle modification significantly reduces features of nonalcoholic steatohepatitis. Gastroenterology 2015;149(2):367–78.e365 [quiz: e314-365]].
33. Kalra S, Kapoor N, Kota S, et al. Person-centred Obesity Care - Techniques, Thresholds, Tools and Targets. Eur Endocrinol 2020;16(1):11–3.
34. Varkaneh HK, Poursoleiman F, Al Masri MK, et al. Low fat diet versus low carbohydrate diet for management of non-alcohol fatty liver disease: a systematic review. Front Nutr 2022;9:987921.

35. Haigh L, Kirk C, El Gendy K, et al. The effectiveness and acceptability of mediterranean diet and calorie restriction in non-alcoholic fatty liver disease (NAFLD): a systematic review and meta-analysis. Clin Nutr 2022;41(9):1913–31.

36. Różański G, Pheby D, Newton JL, et al. Effect of different types of intermittent fasting on biochemical and anthropometric parameters among patients with metabolic-associated fatty liver disease (MAFLD)-a systematic review. Nutrients 2021;14(1):91.

37. Yin C, Li Z, Xiang Y, et al. Effect of intermittent fasting on non-alcoholic fatty liver disease: systematic review and meta-analysis. Front Nutr 2021;8:709683.

38. Scragg J, Avery L, Cassidy S, et al. Feasibility of a very low calorie diet to achieve a sustainable 10% weight loss in patients with nonalcoholic fatty liver disease. Clin Transl Gastroenterol 2020;11(9):e00231.

39. Ramasamy S, Joseph M, Jiwanmall SA, et al. obesity indicators and health-related quality of life - insights from a cohort of morbidly obese, middle-aged South Indian women. Eur Endocrinol 2020;16(2):148–51.

40. Zhou BJ, Huang G, Wang W, et al. Intervention effects of four exercise modalities on nonalcoholic fatty liver disease: a systematic review and Bayesian network meta-analysis. Eur Rev Med Pharmacol Sci 2021;25(24):7687–97.

41. Hong F, Liu Y, Lebaka VR, et al. Effect of exercise training on serum transaminases in patients with nonalcoholic fatty liver disease: a systematic review and meta-analysis. Front Physiol 2022;13:894044.

42. Jeeyavudeen MS, Khan SK, Fouda S, et al. Management of metabolic-associated fatty liver disease: the diabetology perspective. World J Gastroenterol 2023;29(1):126–43.

43. Zafar Y, Rashid AM, Siddiqi AK, et al. Effect of novel glucose lowering agents on non-alcoholic fatty liver disease: a systematic review and meta-analysis. Clin Res Hepatol Gastroenterol 2022;46(7):101970.

44. Kalra S, Bhattacharya S, Kapoor N. Contemporary classification of glucagon-like peptide 1 receptor agonists (GLP1RAs). Diabetes Ther 2021;12(8):2133–47.

45. Kalra S, Arora S, Kapoor N. Classification of non-insulin glucose lowering drugs. J Pak Med Assoc 2022;72(1):181–2.

46. Cusi K, Isaacs S, Barb D, et al. American association of clinical endocrinology clinical practice guideline for the diagnosis and management of nonalcoholic fatty liver disease in primary care and endocrinology clinical settings: co-sponsored by the American association for the study of liver diseases (AASLD). Endocr Pract 2022;28(5):528–62.

47. Kalra S, Bhattacharya S, Kapoor N. Glucagon-like peptide 1 receptor agonists (GLP1RA) and sodium-glucose co-transporter-2 inhibitors (SGLT2i): making a pragmatic choice in diabetes management. J Pak Med Assoc 2022;72(5):989–90.

48. Boutari C, Pappas PD, Anastasilakis D, et al. Statins' efficacy in non-alcoholic fatty liver disease: a systematic review and meta-analysis. Clin Nutr 2022;41(10):2195–206.

49. Alcala M, Calderon-Dominguez M, Serra D, et al. Short-term vitamin E treatment impairs reactive oxygen species signaling required for adipose tissue expansion, resulting in fatty liver and insulin resistance in obese mice. PLoS One 2017;12(10):e0186579.

50. Wang H, Wang L, Cheng Y, et al. Efficacy of orlistat in non-alcoholic fatty liver disease: a systematic review and meta-analysis. Biomed Rep 2018;9(1):90–6.

51. Madhu SV, Kapoor N, Das S, et al. ESI clinical practice guidelines for the evaluation and management of obesity In India. Indian J Endocrinol Metab 2022;26(4): 295–318.
52. Jaleel R, Kapoor N, Kalra S. Endoscopic intragastric balloon: a novel therapy for weight loss. J Pak Med Assoc 2022;72(7):1444–6.
53. Lee SM, Kwak SH, Koo JN, et al. Non-alcoholic fatty liver disease in the first trimester and subsequent development of gestational diabetes mellitus. Diabetologia 2019;62(2):238–48.
54. Mosca A, De Cosmi V, Parazzini F, et al. The role of genetic predisposition, programing during fetal life, family conditions, and post-natal diet in the development of pediatric fatty liver disease. J Pediatr 2019;211:72–7.e74.
55. Muzurović E, Rizzo M, Mikhailidis DP. Obesity and nonalcoholic fatty liver disease in type 1 diabetes mellitus patients. J Diabet Complications 2022;36(12):108359.
56. de Vries M, El-Morabit F, van Erpecum KJ, et al. Non-alcoholic fatty liver disease: identical etiologic factors in patients with type 1 and type 2 diabetes. Eur J Intern Med 2022;100:77–82.
57. de Vries M, Westerink J, El-Morabit F, et al. Prevalence of non-alcoholic fatty liver disease (NAFLD) and its association with surrogate markers of insulin resistance in patients with type 1 diabetes. Diabetes Res Clin Pract 2022;186:109827.
58. Barros BSV, Monteiro FC, Terra C, et al. Prevalence of non-alcoholic fatty liver disease and its associated factors in individuals with type 1 diabetes: a cross-sectional study in a tertiary care center in Brazil. Diabetol Metab Syndrome 2021;13(1):33.
59. Sae-Wong J, Chaopathomkul B, Phewplung T, et al. The Prevalence of Nonalcoholic Fatty Liver Disease and Its Risk Factors in Children and Young Adults with Type 1 Diabetes Mellitus. J Pediatr 2021;230:32–7.e31.
60. Memaj P, Jornayvaz FR. Non-alcoholic fatty liver disease in type 1 diabetes: prevalence and pathophysiology. Front Endocrinol 2022;13:1031633.
61. Ajmera V, Cepin S, Tesfai K, et al. A prospective study on the prevalence of NAFLD, advanced fibrosis, cirrhosis and hepatocellular carcinoma in people with type 2 diabetes. J Hepatol 2022;471–8.
62. McPherson S, Hardy T, Henderson E, et al. Evidence of NAFLD progression from steatosis to fibrosing-steatohepatitis using paired biopsies: implications for prognosis and clinical management. J Hepatol 2015;62(5):1148–55.
63. Simon TG, Roelstraete B, Sharma R, et al. Cancer risk in patients with biopsy-confirmed nonalcoholic fatty liver disease: a population-based cohort study. Hepatology 2021;74(5):2410–23.
64. Tang A, Ng CH, Phang PH, et al. Comparative burden of metabolic dysfunction in lean NAFLD vs Non-lean NAFLD - a systematic review and meta-analysis. Clin Gastroenterol Hepatol 2022;00669–3.
65. Kapoor N, Lotfaliany M, Sathish T, et al. Prevalence of normal weight obesity and its associated cardio-metabolic risk factors - results from the baseline data of the Kerala diabetes prevention program (KDPP). PLoS One 2020;15(8):e0237974.
66. Kapoor N, Furler J, Paul TV, et al. Normal weight obesity: an underrecognized problem in individuals of South Asian descent. Clin Ther 2019;41(8):1638–42.
67. Kapoor N, Lotfaliany M, Sathish T, et al. Effect of a peer-led lifestyle intervention on individuals with normal weight obesity: insights from the Kerala diabetes prevention program. Clin Ther 2020;42(8):1618–24.
68. Xu R, Pan J, Zhou W, et al. Recent advances in lean NAFLD. Biomed Pharmacother 2022;153:113331.

Metabolic-Associated Fatty Liver Disease and the Gut Microbiota

Thomas M. Barber, MA (Hons Cantab), MBBS, DPhil (Oxon), FRCP, FHEA, FAoP[a,b,*], Petra Hanson, MBChB, MRCP, FHEA, PhD[a,b], Martin O. Weickert, MD, FRCP[a,b,c]

KEYWORDS

- Obesity • Metabolic-associated fatty liver disease • Gut microbiota

KEY POINTS

- Driven by the burgeoning global obesity problem, metabolic-associated fatty liver disease (MAFLD) is now the most common cause of chronic liver disease, with a global prevalence of ≥25%.
- Much twenty-first century chronic ill-health likely has its pathogenic origins within the dysbiotic milieu of the gastrointestinal tract.
- The gut–liver axis (GLA) is a nutrient-based highway between the gut and the liver via the portal vein and provides a direct conduit for the gut microbiota and gut-derived metabolic by-products (GDMBs) to interact with the liver.
- Key GLA-related factors contribute towards the development of MAFLD, including the gut microbiota, host inflammatory response, integrity of the gut mucosal wall, and GDMBs that include secondary bile acids, ethanol, and trimethylamine.
- Possible preventive and therapeutic strategies for MAFLD that target the gut microbiota and GLA include probiotics, prebiotics, bile acids, short-chain fatty acids, fecal microbiota transplantation, carbon nanoparticles, and bacteriophages.

Invited Review Article for "Endocrinology and Metabolism Clinics of North America."
[a] Division of Biomedical Sciences, Warwick Medical School, Clinical Sciences Research Laboratories, University Hospitals Coventry and Warwickshire, Clifford Bridge Road, Coventry CV2 2DX, UK; [b] Warwickshire Institute for the Study of Diabetes, Endocrinology and Metabolism, University Hospitals Coventry and Warwickshire, Clifford Bridge Road, Coventry CV2 2DX, UK; [c] Centre of Applied Biological & Exercise Sciences, Faculty of Health & Life Sciences, Coventry University, Coventry CV1 5FB, UK
* Corresponding author. Division of Biomedical Sciences, Warwick Medical School, Clinical Sciences Research Laboratories, University Hospitals Coventry and Warwickshire, Clifford Bridge Road, Coventry CV2 2DX, UK.
E-mail address: T.Barber@warwick.ac.uk

Endocrinol Metab Clin N Am 52 (2023) 485–496
https://doi.org/10.1016/j.ecl.2023.01.004
0889-8529/23/© 2023 Elsevier Inc. All rights reserved.

endo.theclinics.com

INTRODUCTION

Metabolic dysfunction, including most notably type 2 diabetes mellitus (T2D), forms a major component of obesity-associated morbidity and mortality.[1] Insulin resistance and associated hyperinsulinemia, oxidative stress, and a chronic inflammatory milieu underlie such obesity-related metabolic dysfunction, and indeed much obesity-related chronic disease generally.[2] Obesity-associated T2D often coexists with other dysmetabolic conditions that include hypertension, dyslipidemia, and obstructive sleep apnea (OSA).[1] Within this obesity-associated dysmetabolic realm, metabolic-associated fatty liver disease (MAFLD) looms prominently as a key contributor to the pathogenesis of obesity-associated metabolic dysfunction through its close association with insulin resistance and dyslipidemia.[3]

Driven by the burgeoning global obesity problem, MAFLD is now the most common cause of chronic liver disease, with a global prevalence of $\geq 25\%$ and a leading cause of cirrhosis and hepatocellular carcinoma.[4,5] MAFLD is characterized by the accumulation of triglycerides within hepatocytes in non-alcohol users.[6] MAFLD can progress to non-alcoholic steatohepatitis (NASH) in around 10% of patients through complex lipotoxic pathways that implicate mitochondrial and lysosomal dysfunction and stress within the endoplasmic reticulum.[7] Although the pathogenesis of MAFLD is complex and incompletely understood, this likely implicates an array of environmental factors (including diet, lifestyle, physical fitness, sleep sufficiency, and stress) interacting with a background of genetic susceptibility.[8] To add to this gene-environment complexity, in recent years our understanding of the pathogenesis of MAFLD has been transformed by a renewed understanding of the role of the gut microbiota in mediating interactions within the gut–liver axis (GLA). In this narrative review, we provide an overview of the gut microbiota in the development of MAFLD, mediated via the GLA. We explore the therapeutic implications for MAFLD of modifying the gut microbiota composition and targeting the GLA, and the future directions of this promising and emerging field.

The Gut Microbiota

The human microbiota consists of foreign (primarily prokaryotic) cells and occupies multiple locations including the skin and urogenital tract, and most notably the gastrointestinal tract (with approximately 70% of the microbiota inside the colon).[9] Compared with their eukaryotic counterparts, prokaryotic cells, and viruses are much smaller. Therefore, despite their collective and relatively low weight and volume, the gut microbiota out-number our own host cells, with estimates of 100 trillion microbes.[5,10,11] However, only approximately 1000 human-based microbiota have actually been identified to date.[9] Although mostly anaerobic, the precise composition of the gut microbiota is unique to each individual and manifests heterogeneity between individuals. Furthermore, the gut microbiota is influenced by multiple factors that include the site within the gut, age, and lifestyle factors such as physical activity, stress, and importantly, diet.[5]

Our gut microbiota, through coevolution with us over hundreds of millions of years,[10,11] plays an essential role in normal immune development and functioning. Indeed, much twenty-first century chronic ill-health likely has its pathogenic origins within the dysbiotic milieu of the gastrointestinal tract, as a harbinger of aberrant immunological development and functioning.[10,11] Most of our insights into the gut microbiota (and its potential role in human health and disease) stem from evidence derived from rodent-based studies that tend to focus on just one or a collection of gut microbes.[11] However, we should exercise caution in extrapolating insights from rodent-based studies to humans, and we should be cognizant that just as with any organ system, the gut microbiota functions as a whole and includes myriad interactions both between microbes and between microbes and their host. Future research should focus more on human-based studies and extend correlations between individual microbiota and biomarkers to a more holistic approach that considers the impact of the entire gut microbiome (as a functioning unit) on the positioning of its host within the health-disease spectrum. Such an approach will require a more refined and objective definition of the status of the gut microbiota, perhaps as a graded score of the gut microbiota "healthiness" rather than the current use of the dichotomized and rather vague umbrella terms, "eubiosis" and "dysbiosis." We need to explore how the gut microbiota (in its eubiosis-dysbiosis spectral states) interact with us as its host, and vice versa. Such interactions are mediated via the GLA.

The Gut–Liver Axis

Given the separateness of the gut microbiota from the host cells, it is important to explore the mechanisms by which these two entities interact and influence each other. Perhaps unsurprisingly, given the central regulation of appetite, metabolism, mood, and overall well-being, there are close interlinks between the gut microbiota and the brain, mediated via the "gut–brain axis" (GBA). Although beyond the scope of this review, these interactions operate through diverse mechanisms that include neural and hormonal signals, and direct effects of the microbiota and gut-derived metabolic by-products (GDMBs).[12] In addition to the GBA, the gut microbiota interacts with its host through other pathways, most notably the GLA which is particularly relevant for the pathogenesis of MAFLD.

In its broader sense, the GLA is well-characterized and understood.[13] Indeed, the assimilation of nutrients (and detoxification of ingested toxins) as a key role of the liver stems directly from the existence of the GLA. Given the central role of the liver in nutrient handling, it is hardly surprising that a majority (70%) of the liver's blood flow is supplied by the portal vein.[5] However, this direct nutrient-based highway between the gut and the liver via the portal vein also provides a direct conduit for the gut microbiota and GDMBs to interact with the liver. As such, the GLA limits the systemic dissemination of microbes and toxins beyond the liver and enables its function to extend well beyond mere nutrient processing.[5] Importantly, the GLA is bidirectional. In addition to the gut microbiota and GDMBs having direct access to and effects on the liver, bile acids (BAs) and antibodies (each derived from the liver) also have direct access to and effects on the gut microbiota (outlined in **Fig. 1**).[13] Indeed, the liver-coordinated control of the gut microbiota is central to the overall homeostasis and proper functioning of the GLA,[13] which is also influenced by myriad other factors that include the host genetic background and the host interactions with its environment (such as diet and other aspects of lifestyle).[5]

The Gut Microbiota and Gut–Liver Axis in the Pathogenesis of Metabolic-Associated Fatty Liver Disease

A rationale for considering an important role of the gut microbiota in the development of MAFLD (and NASH) stems from the influence of the gut microbiota on the digestion and the absorption of nutrients, and the observation that certain gut microbiota species that are transplanted fecally in rodent-based studies induce obesity.[14] Given the association of MAFLD with obesity, the gut microbiota known to associate with obesity[5] may also overlap somewhat with MAFLD. Furthermore, the gut microbiota influences the development and homeostasis of immunity within the host, and the

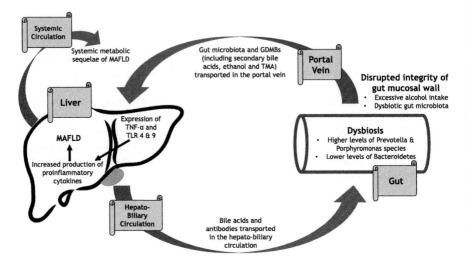

Fig. 1. Overview of the gut microbiota and GLA in the pathogenesis of MAFLD.

production of gut hormones (such as glucagon-like peptide 1 [GLP1]) that modify overall host metabolism.[14]

Compared with healthy controls, people with MAFLD seem to have higher levels of *Prevotella* and *Porphyromonas* species and a lower level of *Bacteroidetes* within their gut microbiota.[5,14] Furthermore, the development of MAFLD seems to depend on the expression within the host of tumor necrosis factor-alpha (TNF-α) receptor and toll-like receptors (TLR) 4 or 9, that in turn likely mediate the hepatic inflammatory response to translocated gut microbiota and/or GDMBs.[5,14] Beyond the type of gut microbiota and host inflammatory response, other key GLA-related factors contribute towards the development of MAFLD, including the integrity of the gut mucosal wall (and the harmful effects of alcohol) and specific GDMBs that include secondary BAs, ethanol, and trimethylamine (TMA).[13]

Integrity of the gut mucosal wall: The functioning of the GLA is influenced by the integrity and intactness of the gut mucosal wall and factors that influence gut mucosal integrity such as the mucus lining of the gut wall. Disruption of the gut mucosal wall can have grave implications for the GLA, with the translocation of gut microbiota into the liver. Indeed, cirrhosis is associated with damage to the gut mucosal wall, including impairments of epithelial, vascular, and immune barriers, associated with profound alterations of the gut microbiota.[13] In eubiosis, small numbers of gut microbiota and GDMBs enter the liver via the portal vein and are mostly eliminated by Kupffer cells. The permeability of the intestinal mucosal barrier (and therefore propensity of bacterial translocation from the gut to the liver) is influenced by multiple physiological protectors that include the mucous layer, tight junctions within the intestinal epithelium, and antimicrobial peptides.[15] Eubiosis promotes an intact intestinal mucosal barrier. Conversely, dysbiotic gut microbiota associates and often coexists with a compromised and permeable intestinal mucosal barrier, resulting at least in part from reduced production of long-chain fatty acids (that in turn promote the growth of commensal Lactobacilli and maintain the gut mucosal wall).[16] Dysbiosis coexisting with a compromised gut mucosal wall can result in exposure of the hepatocytes, Kupffer, and stellate cells to gut microbes and GDMBs (via the portal vein) and hepatic production of proinflammatory cytokines with subsequent development of MAFLD and NASH.[5,17]

Excessive alcohol intake disrupts the GLA at multiple levels, including the gut mucosal wall (including the intestinal epithelial cell tight junction), mucus barrier, antimicrobial peptide production, enhanced inflammatory milieu within the liver, and adverse impact on the gut microbiota itself.[13] Accordingly, alcohol-induced disruption of the GLA represents an important risk factor for both the development of liver disease and dysbiosis with implications for the development of multiple chronic diseases. When the gut-mucosal barrier is compromised by intestinal inflammation (often in the context of dysbiosis), or indeed by other factors like alcohol,[18] large numbers of gut microbiota translocate to the liver, with enhanced activation of Kupffer cells and hepatic stellate cells.[5] Lipopolysaccharides (LPS) represent one particular "bacteria-derived factor" that activates these hepatic cells via binding to TLR 4, with subsequent inflammatory reactions and liver damage.[5]

Secondary bile acids: BAs are produced from cholesterol within the liver and facilitate the absorption of dietary lipids and fat-soluble vitamins.[15,19] Broadly, BAs are classified as primary (synthesized by the liver and accounting for 70% to 80% of the total BA pool), or secondary (primary BAs that are modified by the gut microbiota).[15] BAs are further subclassified according to their conjugation status and hydrophobicity, with considerable potential for heterogeneity in the functioning of BAs (including digestion and nuclear receptor binding).[15] BAs play a key role in mediating interactions between the gut and the liver, including the maintenance of the enterohepatic circulation and intestinal mucosal integrity. Furthermore, dysregulation of BA signaling may contribute to chronic liver diseases such as MAFLD through inflammatory and fibrotic processes.[15]

Most BAs undergo recycling via the enterohepatic circulation, with around 5% of circulating BAs lost in the feces.[15,20] The Farnesoid X receptor (FXR) represents a key mediator of the effects of BAs on the GLA. FXR is a nuclear hormone receptor for BAs, and regulates numerous downstream signaling cascades that include the peroxisome proliferator-activated receptors (PPARs).[15] Other receptor targets of BAs include the Takeda G protein-coupled receptor-5 (TGR5) and the vitamin D receptor.[15] One key mechanism whereby BAs can influence MAFLD development and metabolic health more generally (including glucose, lipid, and cholesterol metabolism) is through the stimulated release of GLP1 from intestinal L-cells via the stimulation of TGR5 receptors as shown in a murine model.[21,22]

Ethanol: The progression of MAFLD to NASH may be influenced by ethanol-producing microbiota.[5] In one study on the composition of the gut microbiota in obese and healthy children and adolescents (determined by 16S ribosomal RNA pyrosequencing), there was an increased representation of alcohol-producing gut bacteria in the NASH participants.[14] A gut microbiome that is rich in ethanol-producing *Escherichia* could represent a driver for the development of MAFLD and NASH in obesity.[14]

TMA: TMA is a GDMB, produced by the gut microbiota during the metabolism of methylamine-containing nutrients, including lecithin, L-carnitine, and choline.[23] Following its delivery to the liver via the portal vein, TMA is further processed to trimethylamine N-oxide (TMAO) by hepatic flavin monooxygenases.[23] There seems to be a correlation between plasma levels of TMAO and both the risk of cardiovascular events and the prevalence of cardiovascular disease in humans.[23,24] Furthermore, in rodent-based models, the gut microbial capacity for the production of TMA seems to influence the size of aortic atherosclerotic lesions.[23] Further rodent-based data supporting a possible role for TMA as a cardiovascular risk factor originates from a *Fmo3* knockdown model, in which reduced atherosclerotic lesions occur.[23,25] (FMO3 is the primary enzyme that converts TMA to TMAO, and itself is regulated by BAs via the FXR receptor).[23] However, associations between levels of TMA and atherosclerotic lesions (derived mainly from rodent studies) are inconsistent and therefore contentious.[23] Future studies should explore possible direct hepatic effects of TMA, including as a potential pathogenic factor for MAFLD, and possible interlinks between BAs and TMA metabolism in the pathogenesis of MAFLD.

Metabolic-Associated Fatty Liver Disease and Therapeutic Implications of the Gut Microbiota and the Gut–Liver Axis

In this section, we explore potential preventive and therapeutic strategies for MAFLD that target the gut microbiota and GLA, including the use of probiotics, prebiotics, antibiotics, BAs, and the FXR, short-chain fatty acids, fecal microbiota transplantation (FMT), carbon nanoparticles, and bacteriophages (summarized in **Table 1**).

Probiotics: Probiotics are live microorganisms intended to have health benefits when consumed or applied to the body. The ingestion of probiotics (including *Lactobacillus*, *Bifidobacterium*, and *Streptococcus*) provides a possible strategy to modify the gut microbiota, and therefore potentially modify the pathogenesis of MAFLD. Engineered probiotics could also be designed to consume toxic metabolites released by the gut microbiota, with conversion into nontoxic chemicals.[13] Animal-based models of NASH using probiotics have shown promising results. Use of the probiotic, "VSL#3" reduced fatty deposits within the liver and associated damage to the liver parenchyma and improved serum alanine aminotransferase (ALT) levels.[5,26] Human-based studies are limited by small sample sizes and potential confounding from lifestyle effects, including diet and exercise.[5] However, despite these limitations, data were reported from four randomized-controlled trials (RCTs) which revealed that probiotic therapy significantly reduced serum levels of ALT,[27–30] but liver steatosis improved in only two of these trials.[29,30] In a meta-analysis of these four RCTs, probiotic therapy was associated with significant improvements in insulin sensitivity (homeostasis model assessment of insulin resistance), and significant reductions in serum levels of TNF-α, aminotransferases, total cholesterol, and high-density lipoprotein (HDL) cholesterol.[31] In a more recent systematic review and meta-analysis of the literature, probiotics were shown to reduce serum ALT and AST levels in people with MAFLD.[16,32,33] Combined, these data provide proof of concept for the potential therapeutic benefits of probiotics, worthy of further scientific scrutiny in larger and better-powered RCTs in multiple and diverse population groups.

Prebiotics: A prebiotic is a substance that promotes the growth of beneficial intestinal microorganisms. A useful analogy here is the use of fertilizer within the soil to promote the growth of plants within a garden. Dietary fiber (the nondigestible component of plant-based foods) provides a natural form of prebiotic.[34] The ingestion of prebiotic supplements such as inulin and oligofructose in people with MAFLD and T2D has been shown to improve serum transaminase activity and glycemic and lipid profiles.[35–37] Furthermore, an RCT on the metabolic effects of synbiotics (a combination of probiotics with prebiotics) combined with lifestyle intervention resulted in significant reductions in hepatic steatosis and fibrosis, and improved markers of glycemia, lipid profile, and inflammatory mediators.[38] As with probiotics, the potential metabolic benefits of prebiotics, including their combination with probiotics as synbiotics should be explored further.

Antibiotics: The role of bacterial translocation between the gut and liver in the development and progression of chronic liver conditions like MAFLD provides a rationale for antibiotic prophylaxis to reduce intestinal bacterial overgrowth, thereby protecting the liver from bacterial exposure and its deleterious pathogenic consequences.[15] However, prophylactic antibiotic administration does not usually form part of the conventional management of MAFLD due to a relative lack of supportive data. Furthermore, the

Table 1
Potential preventive and therapeutic strategies for metabolic-associated fatty liver disease that target the gut microbiota and gut–liver axis

Strategy	Rationale	Rodent-Based Data	Human-Based Data
Probiotics	Live microorganisms to modify gut microbiota	VSL#3 reduced fatty deposits within the liver and improved serum ALT	RCTs and meta-analysis: Improved serum ALT, insulin sensitivity, and lipids
Prebiotics	Promotion of growth of beneficial gut microbiota	—	Improved serum transaminase activity and glycemic/lipid profiles
Antibiotics	Reduces overgrowth of the gut microbiota	—	Microbial resistance to antibiotics precludes this as a viable option
Bile acids	Reduces translocation of gut microbiota to liver	Reduced gut microbial overgrowth and translocation to liver	—
SCFA	Provides energy substrate for colonic epithelium	—	Immunomodulatory and anti-inflammatory properties
FMT	Transformation of the gut microbiota to eubiosis	Altered microbiota and alleviated steatohepatitis and endotoxemia	Either transient or no improvement in insulin sensitivity
Carbon nanoparticles	Detoxifies by-products of the gut microbiota	Yaq-001 attenuated production of ROS and altered microbiota	Trial of Yaq-001 ongoing
Bacteriophages	Promotes eubiosis through "phage cocktail"	—	Trial in primary sclerosing cholangitis ongoing

Abbreviations: ALT, alanine transaminase; FMT, fecal microbiota transplantation; GDMBs, gut-derived metabolic by-products; GLA, gut–liver axis; MAFLD, metabolic-associated fatty liver disease; RCT, randomized controlled trial; ROS, reactive oxygen species; SCFA, short chain fatty acid; TLR, toll-like receptor; TMA, trimethylamine; TNF-α, tumor necrosis factor-alpha; "VSL#3," a probiotic; "Yaq-001," a synthetic non-absorbable carbon that adsorbs bacterial toxins.

burgeoning problem of antibiotic resistance globally[39] relegates the use of antibiotic use as an unlikely future treatment option for MAFLD.

BAs and the FXR: As mediators of the GLA, orally administered BAs (acting via the FXR receptor) provide a therapeutic opportunity for MAFLD via modulation of the GLA. In a mouse model in which cirrhosis was induced, there was gross impairment of the gut muco-epithelial barrier (promoting gut bacterial translocation).[40] However, the impaired gut mucosal wall was modulated by FXR-agonist therapies that also reduced the gut bacterial translocation to the liver via the portal-venous route.[40] In a separate rodent model of cirrhosis, oral administration of BAs reduced intestinal bacterial overgrowth and bacterial translocation,[15] with these effects likely mediated via the FXR receptor.[15,41] Furthermore, in a mouse model of colitis, treatment with the FXR agonist, obeticholic acid (OCA), improved intestinal barrier integrity.[15,42] However, we lack human-based data on the potential therapeutic benefits of BAs in MAFLD.[15,19]

Short-chain fatty acids: Within the human colon, the digestion of dietary fiber (including nondigestible complex carbohydrates, cellulose, and plant polysaccharides) occurs through the action of fermentation by the gut microbiota.[5] This process enables the gut microbiota to yield energy to facilitate their own growth, and the release of a GDMB termed "short-chain fatty acids" (SCFAs).[5,11] These organic fatty acids have health-promoting properties for the human host that includes butyrate acting as an energy substrate for the colonic epithelium, and propionate and acetate as energy substrates for the peripheral tissues.[5] SCFAs may also have immunomodulatory and anti-inflammatory properties and influence the hepatic control of carbohydrate and lipid metabolism.[5,43] The existing data on the potential health benefits of SCFAs promote their therapeutic potential in the management and/or prevention of MAFLD. Currently, we lack human-based data to support such an approach. Furthermore, SCFAs may simply increase energy intake without playing a major role in improved metabolic health.[44,45] However, the encouragement of a high-fiber diet should form an integral part of the management and prevention of MAFLD.[34]

FMT: Currently within the National Health Service (NHS) of the United Kingdom, the use of FMT is reserved solely for the management of patients suffering from intractable colonic colonization with *Clostridium difficile*.[46] Based on data from rodent studies, FMT has the potential as a future treatment option for MAFLD. In a high-fat diet-induced model of steatohepatitis in mice, FMT for 8 weeks corrected disturbances in the gut microbiota (including an elevated abundance of *Lactobacillus* and *Christensenellaceae*).[47] Furthermore, in mice that received FMT there was the alleviation of steatohepatitis (with a significant reduction in intrahepatic lipid accumulation and pro-inflammatory cytokines), improved intestinal tight junction protein "ZO-1," and reduced endotoxemia.[47] However, early reported human-based studies on the metabolic effects of FMT have been disappointing, with only transient improvements in insulin sensitivity and without appreciable improvements in other clinical parameters.[16] A more recent assessment of the metabolic effects of a fecal capsule in obese adults showed no significant improvement in insulin sensitivity or body composition.[16,48] The conflicting data on FMT between rodents and humans may be partly explained by behavioral differences (such as the practice of coprophagia), that highlight important limitations of rodent-based models in this context.[49,50]

Carbon nanoparticles: An alternative therapeutic strategy to modification of the gut microbiota through FMT includes detoxification of the toxic byproducts of the gut microbiota, thereby limiting their pathogenic effects within the liver via the GLA. Yaq-001 is a synthetic nonabsorbable carbon that adsorbs bacterial toxins. In a rodent model of Secondary Biliary Cirrhosis, Yaq-001 significantly attenuated LPS-induced production of reactive oxygen species within monocytes and altered the ratio of Firmicutes and Bacteroidetes.[13] A human-based study of Yaq-001 is currently ongoing.[13]

Bacteriophages: Bacteriophages are viruses that infect and kill bacteria.[13] Therapeutically, bacteriophages can be used to target infectious bacteria. However, an alternate therapeutic strategy involves the development of "phage cocktails" that target specific bacteria within the gut microbiome, to diminish and possibly eliminate those strains that promote dysbiosis while maintaining the healthy gut microbiota.[13] A human-based study on the use of bacteriophage treatment for patients with Primary Sclerosing Cholangitis is ongoing.[13]

SUMMARY AND FUTURE DIRECTIONS

MAFLD is now the most common cause of chronic liver disease, affecting one in four of the world's population, and a leading cause of cirrhosis.[4,5] MAFLD often develops insidiously and asymptomatically in those who gain weight in the context of an underlying genetic predisposition. Based on the evidence outlined, we argue for a seachange in our perspectives on MAFLD as a key linchpin in the complex development of metabolic dysfunction, and as an important gateway and portal between the gut microbiota and the overall metabolic status of the host, mediated via the GLA. As such, MAFLD should be considered as a condition that is influenced in its pathogenesis by the healthiness of the gut microbiota, and the status of the GLA (including the intactness of the gut mucosal wall). Outstanding human-based research questions include the role of the gut microbiota and other GLA-related factors in the development of MAFLD, and optimal preventive, therapeutic, and screening strategies (such as probiotics, prebiotics, synbiotics, and FMT). This will require robust, powerful, and well-validated RCTs, performed in diverse populations. Novel treatment and preventive approaches for MAFLD should focus on improving the healthiness of the gut microbiota and optimizing the proper functioning of the GLA, including avoidance of excessive weight gain through the usual principles of a healthy lifestyle, a healthy and high-fiber diet, and avoidance of excessive alcohol intake. In essence, we need to nurture our gut microbiota to enable our gut microbiota to nurture our GLA, our liver, and us.

CLINICS CARE POINTS

- In the clinical assessment of obesity, it is important to screen for the presence of metabolic-associated fatty liver disease (MAFLD) through liver function tests and where necessary appropriate imaging studies. Other risk factors such as hypertension, dysglycemia, and dyslipidemia should also be screened for.

- It should be noted that the development of MAFLD is often gradual and insidious, and frequently asymptomatic. In patients diagnosed with MAFLD, health care professionals should take the time to explain its development and clinical implications empathically and encourage the adoption of a healthy lifestyle.

- Currently, we lack specific targeted therapies for MAFLD, although novel treatment and preventive approaches to improve the healthiness of our gut microbiota and optimize proper gut–liver axis (GLA) functioning are under development. Our current best advice is to avoid excessive weight gain through the usual principles of a healthy lifestyle (or to lose weight in the context of obesity), adopt and maintain a balanced, healthy, and high-fiber diet, avoid sedentariness and excessive alcohol intake, and optimize stress.

- In short, we need to nurture our gut microbiota to enable our gut microbiota to nurture our GLA, our liver, and us.

CONFLICT OF INTEREST AND FINANCIAL DISCLOSURE

The authors have no conflicts of interest.

FUNDING

This study did not receive any funding.

REFERENCES

1. Pi-Sunyer X. The medical risks of obesity. PGM (Postgrad Med) 2009;121(6):21–33.

2. Fruh SM. Obesity: Risk factors, complications, and strategies for sustainable long-term weight management. Journal of the American Association of Nurse Practitioners 2017;29(S1):S3–14.

3. Sakurai Y., Kubota N., Yamauchi T., et al., Role of insulin resistance in MAFLD, *Int J Mol Sci*, 22 (8), 2021, 4156.

4. Powell EE, Wong VW, Rinella M. Non-alcoholic fatty liver disease. Lancet 2021; 397(10290):2212–24.

5. Minemura M, Shimizu Y. Gut microbiota and liver diseases. World J Gastroenterol 2015;21(6):1691–702.

6. Eslam M, Newsome PN, Sarin SK, et al. A new definition for metabolic dysfunction-associated fatty liver disease: an international expert consensus statement. J Hepatol 2020;73(1):202–9.

7. Geng Y, Faber KN, de Meijer VE, et al. How does hepatic lipid accumulation lead to lipotoxicity in non-alcoholic fatty liver disease? Hepatol Int 2021;15(1):21–35.

8. Jamialahmadi O, Mancina RM, Ciociola E, et al. Exome-wide association study on alanine aminotransferase identifies sequence variants in the GPAM and APOE associated with fatty liver disease. Gastroenterology 2021;160(5): 1634–16346 e7.

9. Mueller NT, Bakacs E, Combellick J, et al. The infant microbiome development: mom matters. Trends Mol Med 2015;21(2):109–17.

10. Qin J, Li R, Raes J, et al. A human gut microbial gene catalogue established by metagenomic sequencing. Nature 2010;464(7285):59–65.

11. Barber T.M., Valsamakis G., Mastorakos G., et al., Dietary influences on the microbiota-gut-brain axis, *Int J Mol Sci*, 22 (7), 2021, 3502.

12. Cryan JF, O'Riordan KJ, Cowan CSM, et al. The microbiota-gut-brain axis. Physiol Rev 2019;99(4):1877–2013.

13. Albillos A, de Gottardi A, Rescigno M. The gut-liver axis in liver disease: Patho-physiological basis for therapy. J Hepatol 2020;72(3):558–77.

14. Zhu L, Baker SS, Gill C, et al. Characterization of gut microbiomes in nonalcoholic steatohepatitis (NASH) patients: a connection between endogenous alcohol and NASH. Hepatology 2013;57(2):601–9.

15. Simbrunner B, Trauner M, Reiberger T. Review article: therapeutic aspects of bile acid signalling in the gut-liver axis. Aliment Pharmacol Ther 2021;54(10): 1243–62.

16. Malnick S.D.H., Fisher D., Somin M., et al., Treating the Metabolic Syndrome by Fecal Transplantation-Current Status, *Biology*, 10 (5), 2021, 447.

17. Mouries J, Brescia P, Silvestri A, et al. Microbiota-driven gut vascular barrier disruption is a prerequisite for non-alcoholic steatohepatitis development. J Hepatol 2019;71(6):1216–28.

18. Seo YS, Shah VH. The role of gut-liver axis in the pathogenesis of liver cirrhosis and portal hypertension. Clin Mol Hepatol 2012;18(4):337–46.

19. Weickert MO, Hattersley JG, Kyrou I, et al. Effects of supplemented isoenergetic diets varying in cereal fiber and protein content on the bile acid metabolic signature and relation to insulin resistance. Nutr Diabetes 2018;8(1):11.

20. Di Ciaula A, Garruti G, Lunardi Baccetto R, et al. Bile acid physiology. Ann Hepatol 2017;16(Suppl. 1: s3–105):s4–14.

21. Katsuma S, Hirasawa A, Tsujimoto G. Bile acids promote glucagon-like peptide-1 secretion through TGR5 in a murine enteroendocrine cell line STC-1. Biochem Biophys Res Commun 2005;329(1):386–90.

22. Thomas C, Gioiello A, Noriega L, et al. TGR5-mediated bile acid sensing controls glucose homeostasis. Cell Metabol 2009;10(3):167–77.

23. Schoeler M, Caesar R. Dietary lipids, gut microbiota and lipid metabolism. Rev Endocr Metab Disord 2019;20(4):461–72.

24. Tang WH, Wang Z, Levison BS, et al. Intestinal microbial metabolism of phosphatidylcholine and cardiovascular risk. N Engl J Med 2013;368(17):1575–84.

25. Miao J, Ling AV, Manthena PV, et al. Flavin-containing monooxygenase 3 as a potential player in diabetes-associated atherosclerosis. Nat Commun 2015;6:6498.

26. Fedorak RN, Madsen KL. Probiotics and prebiotics in gastrointestinal disorders. Curr Opin Gastroenterol 2004;20(2):146–55.

27. Aller R, De Luis DA, Izaola O, et al. Effect of a probiotic on liver aminotransferases in nonalcoholic fatty liver disease patients: a double blind randomized clinical trial. Eur Rev Med Pharmacol Sci 2011;15(9):1090–5.

28. Vajro P, Mandato C, Licenziati MR, et al. Effects of Lactobacillus rhamnosus strain GG in pediatric obesity-related liver disease. J Pediatr Gastroenterol Nutr 2011;52(6):740–3.

29. Malaguarnera M, Vacante M, Antic T, et al. Bifidobacterium longum with fructooligosaccharides in patients with non alcoholic steatohepatitis. Dig Dis Sci 2012;57(2):545–53.

30. Wong VW, Won GL, Chim AM, et al. Treatment of nonalcoholic steatohepatitis with probiotics. A proof-of-concept study. Ann Hepatol 2013;12(2):256–62.

31. Ma YY, Li L, Yu CH, et al. Effects of probiotics on nonalcoholic fatty liver disease: a meta-analysis. World J Gastroenterol 2013;19(40):6911–8.

32. Gilijamse PW, Hartstra AV, Levin E, et al. Treatment with Anaerobutyricum soehngenii: a pilot study of safety and dose-response effects on glucose metabolism in human subjects with metabolic syndrome. NPJ Biofilms Microbiomes 2020;6(1):16.

33. Depommier C, Everard A, Druart C, et al. Supplementation with Akkermansia muciniphila in overweight and obese human volunteers: a proof-of-concept exploratory study. Nat Med 2019;25(7):1096–103.

34. Barber T.M., Kabisch S., Pfeiffer A.F.H., et al., The health benefits of dietary fibre, *Nutrients*, 12 (10), 2020, 3209.

35. Jeznach-Steinhagen A., Ostrowska J., Czerwonogrodzka-Senczyna A., et al., Dietary and pharmacological treatment of nonalcoholic fatty liver disease, *Medicina (Kaunas).*, 55 (5), 2019, 166.

36. Mouzaki M, Comelli EM, Arendt BM, et al. Intestinal microbiota in patients with nonalcoholic fatty liver disease. Hepatology 2013;58(1):120–7.

37. Asemi Z, Khorrami-Rad A, Alizadeh SA, et al. Effects of synbiotic food consumption on metabolic status of diabetic patients: a double-blind randomized crossover controlled clinical trial. Clin Nutr 2014;33(2):198–203.

38. Mofidi F, Poustchi H, Yari Z, et al. Synbiotic supplementation in lean patients with non-alcoholic fatty liver disease: a pilot, randomised, double-blind, placebo-controlled, clinical trial. Br J Nutr 2017;117(5):662–8.

39. Aslam B, Khurshid M, Arshad MI, et al. Antibiotic resistance: one health one world outlook. Front Cell Infect Microbiol 2021;11:771510.

40. Sorribas M, Jakob MO, Yilmaz B, et al. FXR modulates the gut-vascular barrier by regulating the entry sites for bacterial translocation in experimental cirrhosis. J Hepatol 2019;71(6):1126–40.

41. Verbeke L, Farre R, Verbinnen B, et al. The FXR agonist obeticholic acid prevents gut barrier dysfunction and bacterial translocation in cholestatic rats. Am J Pathol 2015;185(2):409–19.

42. Gadaleta RM, van Erpecum KJ, Oldenburg B, et al. Farnesoid X receptor activation inhibits inflammation and preserves the intestinal barrier in inflammatory bowel disease. Gut 2011;60(4):463–72.
43. Maslowski KM, Vieira AT, Ng A, et al. Regulation of inflammatory responses by gut microbiota and chemoattractant receptor GPR43. Nature 2009;461(7268): 1282–6.
44. Weickert MO, Arafat AM, Blaut M, et al. Changes in dominant groups of the gut microbiota do not explain cereal-fiber induced improvement of whole-body insulin sensitivity. Nutr Metab 2011;8:90.
45. Isken F, Klaus S, Osterhoff M, et al. Effects of long-term soluble vs. insoluble dietary fiber intake on high-fat diet-induced obesity in C57BL/6J mice. J Nutr Biochem 2010;21(4):278–84.
46. Kim KO, Gluck M. Fecal microbiota transplantation: an update on clinical practice. Clinical endoscopy 2019;52(2):137.
47. Zhou D, Pan Q, Shen F, et al. Total fecal microbiota transplantation alleviates high-fat diet-induced steatohepatitis in mice via beneficial regulation of gut microbiota. Sci Rep 2017;7(1):1529.
48. Allegretti JR, Kassam Z, Mullish BH, et al. Effects of fecal microbiota transplantation with oral capsules in obese patients. Clin Gastroenterol Hepatol 2020;18(4): 855–863 e2.
49. Weickert MO, Pfeiffer AFH. Impact of dietary fiber consumption on insulin resistance and the prevention of type 2 diabetes. J Nutr 2018;148(1):7–12.
50. Weickert MO, Pfeiffer AF. Metabolic effects of dietary fiber consumption and prevention of diabetes. J Nutr 2008;138(3):439–42.

Metabolic-Associated Fatty Liver Disease and Sarcopenia

Triada Bali, MD, Lampros Chrysavgis, MD, PhDc,
Evangelos Cholongitas, MD, PhD*

KEYWORDS

- MAFLD • Sarcopenia • Insulin resistance • Sarcopenic obesity • Diet
- Physical activity

KEY POINTS

- Metabolic-associated fatty liver disease and sarcopenia often coexist, as they share many pathophysiologic mechanisms.
- Both entities are associated with higher risk for metabolic and other comorbidities.
- There is no approved pharmacotherapy yet.
- Early screening and detection of both the disorders are necessary for appropriate lifestyle modifications to improve health outcomes.

INTRODUCTION

Sarcopenia is defined as a progressive loss of skeletal muscle mass, strength, and function.[1] Sarcopenia is often associated with ageing and frailty and, more recently, has been linked to metabolic syndrome and its manifestations of type 2 diabetes mellitus (T2DM), cardiovascular diseases, and metabolic-associated fatty liver disease (MAFLD).[2,3]

The muscle-liver-adipose tissue axis plays a major role in shaping the body composition.[2] Studies reporting clinical and experimental data imply that sarcopenia and MAFLD are associated with lipotoxicity and ectopic fat storage in the skeletal muscles (myosteatosis) and hepatic parenchyma, respectively.[4] Understanding the possible role of sarcopenia in the progression of MAFLD, and vice versa, is crucial for planning appropriate preventive and therapeutic strategies. Scarcity of data on whether sarcopenia causes MAFLD directly/indirectly or vice versa may lead to inappropriate clinical decisions. Therefore, further studies are needed to investigate the interconnection

First Department of Internal Medicine, General Hospital of Athens "Laiko", Medical School of National and Kapodistrian University of Athens, 17 Agiou Thoma Street, Athens 11527, Greece
* Corresponding author.
E-mail address: cholongitas@yahoo.gr

Endocrinol Metab Clin N Am 52 (2023) 497–508
https://doi.org/10.1016/j.ecl.2023.02.004
0889-8529/23/© 2023 Elsevier Inc. All rights reserved.

between these 2 disorders. In this current review, the authors aim to elaborate the current evidence on this debated issue.

THE INTERLINK BETWEEN SARCOPENIA AND METABOLIC-ASSOCIATED FATTY LIVER DISEASE

MAFLD is currently the main cause of chronic liver disease, affecting 29.8% of people globally.[5] Sarcopenia is also a very common condition, especially in specific population groups, such as the elderly (5%–10%), obese individuals (6%–43%), patients suffering from liver cirrhosis of any cause (40%–70%), as well as in patients with MAFLD (20%).[6,7] Interestingly, a recent study revealed that among patients with chronic hepatitis B, those with MAFLD have lower muscle mass and strength, compared with those without MAFLD (50% vs 21.7%, respectively).[8]

Sarcopenia has been related to advanced MAFLD-associated liver inflammation and fibrosis with a stepwise increase in the prevalence of sarcopenia with severity of liver histological lesions).[9,10] A 7-year Korean cohort study pointed out the effect of muscle maintenance and strengthening on MAFLD resolution.[11] Therefore, it has been suggested that sarcopenia may be a disease modifier of MAFLD, and thus its early detection seems to be crucial.[2] In addition, the presence of sarcopenia seems to increase the cardiovascular risk and mortality in patients with MAFLD by aggravation of atherosclerosis and metabolic alterations regardless of other metabolic factors, such as obesity and insulin resistance (IR).[12,13] These findings were confirmed in a recent study with 3042 participants, which revealed an additive effect of sarcopenia on the determination of cardiovascular disease risk in patients with MAFLD,[14] indicating the adverse impact of sarcopenia on the metabolic consequences and outcome in this group of patients.

CAUSE-EFFECT RELATIONSHIP

Given that the 2 conditions share numerous similar pathophysiological processes, it is unclear whether MAFLD induces sarcopenia or sarcopenia is a promoting factor for MAFLD onset and progression. In the current section the authors aim to provide a short overview of these mechanisms, which are comprehensively illustrated in **Fig. 1**. More precisely, ageing and behavioral parameters are significant risk factors for the development of sarcopenia and MAFLD.[15] The normal process of ageing is a low-grade chronic inflammatory state, characterized by increased cellular senescence, mitochondrial dysfunction, and defective autophagy,[15] and is also associated with detrimental changes in the concentration of major hormones including testosterone, growth hormone (GH), and insulin like growth factor-1 (IGF-1).[16] Testosterone, as an anabolic hormone, has a pivotal role in muscle protein synthesis. Lower levels of testosterone are significantly associated with sarcopenia and sarcopenic obesity (SO), especially among older men.[17] Concurrently, estrogen deficiency in postmenopausal women has been related to higher prevalence of both MAFLD and sarcopenia.[18] Interestingly, low vitamin D levels have been observed in patients with IR, T2DM, dyslipidemia, and other aspects of metabolic dysregulation,[19] as well as in sarcopenic individuals.[3] In addition, a hypercaloric diet with high fructose and saturated or trans-fat consumption[20] and reduced protein intake along with lack of physical exercise[21] can induce MAFLD, obesity, as well as low muscle protein synthesis and sarcopenia.[7,22] The excessive adiposity can result in ectopic fat accumulation in the hepatic parenchyma and skeletal muscle.[3,23]

The progression of MAFLD to significant fibrosis and cirrhosis causes insufficient ammonia decomposition, which in turn results in hyperammonemia.[24] The latter

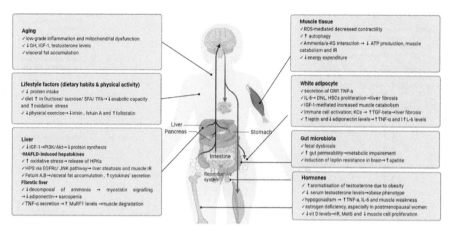

Fig. 1. The major risk factors and pathophysiological mechanisms that contribute to sarcopenia in patients with metabolic-associated fatty liver disease (MAFLD). a-KG, alphaketoglutarate; CRP, C-reactive protein; DNL, de novo lipogenesis; EGFRc, epidermal growth factor receptor c; GH, growth hormone; HPKs, hepatokines; HPS, hepassocin; HSCs, hepatic stellate cells; IGF-1, insulin-like growth factor-1; IL-6, interleukin-6; IR, insulin resistance; JNK, Janus N-terminal kinase; KCs, Kupffer cells; MuRF1, muscle RING-finger protein-1; PI3K, phosphoinositide 3-kinase; SFA, saturated fatty acids; TFA, trans-fatty acids; TGF-beta, transforming growth factor-beta; TNF-α, tumor necrosis factor alpha; vit D, vitamin D.

promotes sarcopenia because the muscle tissue becomes the major organ for ammonia disposal, leading to decreased α-ketoglutarate levels, impaired mitochondrial activity, and lower protein synthesis.[24] Consistent with that, hyperammonemia facilitates the upregulation of myostatin, a major myokine, which markedly hinders satellite cell proliferation in muscle and thereby promotes muscle wasting. In addition, myostatin is thought to reduce adiponectin production, inducing liver and muscle fat accumulation,[25] further enhancing the vicious interorgan crosstalk among liver, muscle, and adipose tissue. In line, low levels of irisin which is another important myokine, seem to be implicated in the development of both MAFLD and sarcopenia, while reduced irisin concentration has been noted in patients with MAFLD and obese individuals compared to lean controls.[26]

MAFLD-associated inflammation drives the secretion of several hepatokines, such as fetuin A and B, selenoprotein P, fibroblast growth factor 21, leukocyte cell–derived chemotaxin 2, and hepassocin.[7,22] Hepassocin is related to liver fat accumulation and IR induction in the skeletal muscle through the epidermal growth factor receptor/c-Jun N-terminal kinases signaling pathway.[7,22] MAFLD-associated inflammation and fibrosis is also involved in muscle catabolism via elevated production of tumor necrosis factor-α,[27] which activates nuclear factor-kB signaling in muscle and drives the upregulation of muscle RING-finger protein-1 promoting muscle degradation and atrophy.[28] Interestingly, recent studies have shown that alterations in gut microbiome are associated with liver histological lesions in individuals with MAFLD[29] and changes in muscle phenotype,[30] pinpointing that MAFLD and sarcopenia share another common denominator. Lastly, those alterations in the intestinal microbiome cause IR in peripheral tissues, the role of which is discussed herein.

The Role of Insulin Resistance

Of clinical importance, insulin plays a key role in the triangular interaction between liver, adipose tissue, and muscle (**Fig. 2**). Physiologically, the binding of insulin to its

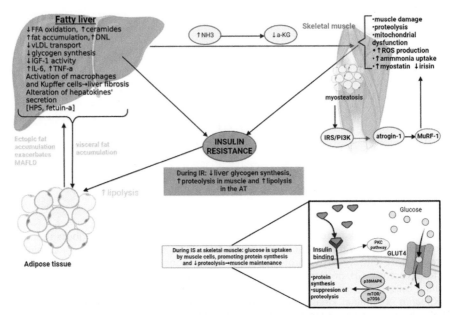

Fig. 2. The impact of insulin resistance on the triangle crosstalk between muscle mass, adipose tissue, and liver. a-KG, alpha ketoglutarate; AT, adipose tissue; DNL, de novo lipogenesis; FFA, free fatty acids; GLUT4, glucose transporter type 4; HPS, hepassocin; IGF-1, insulin growth factor-1; IL-6, interleukin-6; IR, insulin resistance; IRS-1/PI3K, insulin receptor substrates-1/phosphoinositide 3-kinase; IS, insulin sensitivity; MAPK, mitogen-activated protein kinase; mTOR, mammalian target of rapamycin; MuRF-1, muscle RING-finger protein-1; NH3, ammonia; PKC, protein kinase C; ROS, reactive oxygen species; TNF-α, tumour necrosis factor alpha; vLDL, very low-density lipoprotein.

receptors in the muscle cells facilitates the translocation of glucose transporter type 4 (GLUT-4) from the intracellular domain to the plasma membrane to mediate the glucose uptake by the muscle cells. This, in turn, increases the activity of the phosphatidylinositol 3-kinase/Akt and mammalian target of rapamycin signaling pathways, which results in elevated muscle protein synthesis and inhibition of proteolysis.[7,31]

IR promotes proteolysis and muscle catabolism, partially via the induction of the ubiquitin ligase atrogin-1 and the MuRF1 protein.[32] Concurrently, IR induces lipolysis in the adipose tissue, which generates free fatty acids (FFAs) that can be delivered to both liver and muscle, inducing MAFLD and myosteatosis, respectively.[23,33] The reduced lean muscle mass and the muscle fat accumulation further exacerbates IR as well as mitigates the uptake of FFAs by muscle tissue.[33] Their increased delivery to the hepatic parenchyma augments hepatic lipotoxicity, reactive oxygen species (ROS) production, and hepatocyte damage, promoting the vicious cycle of IR and intrahepatic fat accumulation that ultimately leads to the progression of MAFLD to steatohepatitis, fibrosis, and liver cirrhosis.[2,34]

METABOLIC-ASSOCIATED FATTY LIVER DISEASE AND SARCOPENIC OBESITY

SO is characterized by reduced muscle strength and function and obesity (body mass index [BMI] > 30 kg/m², >27.5 kg/m² for Asians).[35] In patients with SO, BMI may be unchanged, but baseline metabolic rate is usually reduced. According to a recent meta-analysis, SO affects 11% of the global population, whereas the prevalence increases to 23.0% in subjects aged 75 years or older.[36] Interestingly, many studies have shown a high prevalence of SO in patients with MAFLD, especially in those with advance stages of fibrosis.[37,38]

It seems that the clinical interactions between sarcopenia and obesity result in higher and additive risk for metabolic dysregulation and more importantly cardiovascular morbidity and mortality compared with sarcopenia or obesity alone.[39,40] At molecular level, SO, similar to sarcopenia, is characterized by loss of motor unit number, reduction in number of both type I and II muscle fibers, as well as decrease in the size of the latter, defined as atrophy.[41] Moreover, the transition of type II muscle fibers to slow type I muscle fibers, which are less insulin sensitive and have higher content of mitochondria constitute another common aspect of sarcopenia and SO.[41] Type I fibers become dysfunctional during ageing and generate ROS enhancing this vicious cycle of muscle damage.[42] Besides the aforementioned changes in skeletal muscle mass, SO is characterized by the additional emergence of obesity, during which fat infiltration into muscle (myosteatosis) is observed.[43]

However, it should be mentioned that the diagnosis of SO may be difficult because of adipose tissue interfering with the evaluation of muscle mass.[43] Nevertheless, prompt diagnosis of SO is crucial, but therapy can be a challenge, as nutritional intervention should aim at losing weight and enhancing muscle mass at the same time.[2]

SCREENING AND DIAGNOSIS (ASSESSING MUSCLE COMPOSITION, STRENGTH, AND PERFORMANCE IN METABOLIC-ASSOCIATED FATTY LIVER DISEASE)

According to the latest updated definition of sarcopenia by the European Working Group on Sarcopenia in Older People (EWGSOP) in 2018, there are 3 basic parameters to be assessed: muscle strength, muscle quantity as well as quality and physical performance.[44]

Muscle Strength

According to the recommended algorithm,[3,44] SARC-F, a simple questionnaire evaluating muscle Strength, Assistance in walking, Rising from a chair, stair Climbing, and experiences with Falls, can be used for patients' screening although its sensitivity is relatively low. A score greater than or equal to 4 is indicative of sarcopenia.[45] If sarcopenia is suspected based on SARC-F or clinical evidence, the next step is to assess muscle strength, which is considered a superior outcome predictor than quantification of muscle mass, based on hand grip test and 30-second chair stand test (30 CST). If low strength is detected (ie, hand grip strength <27 kg in men or <16 kg in women, 30 CST >15 sec), then sarcopenia is thought to be probable, and further assessment and intervention can be initiated.[44] Furthermore, as proposed by guidelines, the evaluation of muscle strength shall be considered as major parameter for the assessment of SO.[46]

Muscle Quantity

To confirm the diagnosis of sarcopenia, other tests for muscle mass evaluation, such as dual energy X-absorptiometry (DEXA), bioelectrical impedance analysis (BIA) as well as lumbar muscle cross-sectional area assessment can be performed. The latter can be evaluated by computed tomography (CT), MRI, or ultrasound.[3] Indices based on DEXA measurement, such as total body lean mass (LM), lean mass index (LMI: LM adjusted for height), appendicular lean mass (ALM), and appendicular lean mass index (ALMI: ALM adjusted for height and BMI) are useful. However, there are some limitations, as fluid retention can cause an overestimation of muscle mass, whereas intramuscular fat, which accounts for 5% to 15% of muscle in obese individuals, cannot be detected.[47] Nevertheless, the current guidelines proposed DEXA as the preferable diagnostic tool for the evaluation of body composition, because of its accuracy, high reproducibility, and its low cost.[46] Muscle mass assessed by BIA has some limitations because several external factors and low reproducibility influence its results and consequently cannot be used properly for patients with MAFLD.[48] CT and MRI-based muscle mass evaluation are easily reproducible but not ideal for screening because of their CT-related radiation exposure and/or high cost.[46] Although there are not still well-established cutoff points for patients with MAFLD, both CT and MRI are considered the "gold standard" to estimate intramuscular fat infiltration.[49] Anthropometric measures, such as triceps skinfold and mid-arm muscle circumference, can be easily and carried out at low cost in patients with MAFLD, even though obesity impact on their accuracy remains unknown. Values less than the 10th percentile of the ones from individuals of the same age and gender are considered diagnostic for sarcopenia.[50]

Muscle Quality and Physical Performance

Once sarcopenia is confirmed, the detection of severe cases can be implemented through physical performance evaluation, using timed up and go test, gait speed test, and short physical performance battery (SPPB).[3] Although an SPPB score less than 8 confirms the diagnosis of poor physical performance in elderly people, no validated cutoff point for patients with MAFLD exists. However, there is a ceiling effect (maximum score of 12/12), which impedes appropriate postinterventions assessment. Liver frailty index is liver specific, overcomes SPPB ceiling effect, and seems to predict the morbidity and mortality with reliable accuracy before and after liver transplantation.[51] A score greater than 4.4 defines sarcopenia, but it has been evaluated only in cirrhotic patients.[22,52]

In conclusion, although screening for sarcopenia as a routine in patients with MAFLD is still controversial, and the definition remains questionable, the identification of sarcopenia may be useful as a potential factor to stratify patients with MAFLD in groups of lower or greater risk for fibrosis progression and mortality, as well as to implement appropriate nutritional interventions and encourage physical activity (enhancement of muscle mass) with beneficial effect in both sarcopenia and MAFLD.[14]

COMPLICATIONS (ESPECIALLY WHEN BOTH ENTITIES COEXIST, INCLUDING CARDIOVASCULAR RISK)

Patients with MAFLD are at a higher risk for hepatocellular carcinoma compared with the general population, even in the absence of cirrhosis due to several pathogenetic mechanisms including IR, elevated levels of ROS, and genetic predisposition.[53] Several studies have also proposed a correlation between MAFLD and other IR-associated metabolic and/or extra-hepatic chronic conditions.[54,55] Nevertheless, the main cause of morbidity and mortality in patients with MAFLD are cardiovascular diseases.[56] It has been noted that there is a great association between MAFLD and atherosclerosis,[54] whereas hyperinsulinemia-induced renin-angiotensin-aldosterone system activation plays an important role in chronic cardiac dysfunction and cardiac stiffness.[57]

The presence of sarcopenia seems to increase the risk for cardiovascular, T2DM-related, cancer, and all-cause mortality in patients with MAFLD[13,58] via modification of metabolic parameters and increases disability and frailty. Regarding cardiovascular complications, sarcopenia is related to mitochondrial dysfunction and an increased release of cytokines, which promote atherosclerosis and heart fibrosis.[59] Interestingly, data from the Korean National Health and Nutrition Examination Surveys (KNHANES) study examining 28,000 individuals showed that MAFLD and sarcopenia additively increase mortality risk independently of liver fibrosis stage.[60] Consistently, a Korean study showed that albuminuria (which is a known independent risk factor for all-cause and cardiovascular mortality) was prevalent among patients with MAFLD and importantly associated with the presence of sarcopenia.[61]

THERAPEUTIC AND LIFESTYLE INTERVENTIONS

Patients with MAFLD should be encouraged to lose weight, and the degree of weight reduction reflects the degree of improvement in liver histology.[62] As implementing strict exercise programs to enhance weight loss is inevitably accompanied by muscle mass loss, high protein intake and low sucrose/fructose consumption is recommended to minimize muscle catabolism.[46] Therefore, calorie restriction and/or weight loss programs in sarcopenic patients should be implemented cautiously and on an individual basis. A combination of resistance and aerobic physical exercise should be added to nutritional intervention in order to maintain muscle mass and strength, which would be helpful for both MAFLD and sarcopenia.[46] Physical activity has a beneficial effect on liver steatosis through higher GLUT4 expression, ameliorating insulin

Table 1
Recommended therapeutic lifestyle approaches and experimental interventions for metabolic-associated fatty liver disease and sarcopenia

	Recommendation
Weight loss	In combination with exercise and a diet rich in proteins so as to maintain muscle mass on an individualized basis
Physical activity	Resistance and aerobic exercises for at least 3–5 sessions per week
Diet	High-quality proteins, Mediterranean diet, low fructose and sucrose consumption, calorie restriction if necessary

Experimental Interventions	Mechanism of Action
Testosterone (in men only)	Anabolic hormone, IGF-1 secretion
Growth hormone replacement	Lipolysis of visceral fat, muscle protein synthesis improvement
GLP-1 receptor agonists	GH/IGF-1 axis activation
ACE inhibitors	Prevention of mitochondrial dysfunction, liver steatosis and fibrogenesis reduction, muscle mass improvement
Myostatin inhibitors	Muscle growth, liver profibrotic proteins suppression
Vitamin D	Insulin sensitivity regulation, reduced inflammation, muscle cell proliferation
Polyunsaturated fatty acids	Lipid metabolism improvement
Creatine	Muscle growth, liver steatosis reduction

Abbreviations: ACE, angiotensin-converting enzyme; GLP-1, glucagon-like peptide-1.

sensitivity and improving hepatic lipid metabolism.[63] Long-term exercise programs can prevent MAFLD progression to advanced fibrosis by improving the phagocytic function of liver Kupffer cells and by attenuating the inflammation and fibrogenesis processes.[64]

Nutritional interventions are also needed in order to achieve weight loss and other health benefits possibly including beneficial alterations in gut microbiota.[65] Patients should be encouraged to have stricter adherence to Mediterranean diet, a well-balanced diet with proven effects on reducing body weight, serum lipids, and ultimately cardiovascular risk.[1,66] Nevertheless, it should be considered that especially during the acute fasting phase, even a small amount of high-quality proteins in every meal is needed in order to inhibit protein catabolism, whereas excessive protein intake can result in an increased risk for IR and T2DM development.[46]

Many pharmaceutical products such as creatine, 5 N-3 polyunsaturated fatty acids, vitamin D, as well as GH and testosterone replacement, which have been studied as a treatment of sarcopenia, are also thought to improve liver steatosis.[3,67,68] Interestingly, a recent clinical trial has revealed that a daily oral dose of testosterone can improve both liver steatosis and body composition in noncirrhotic men with MAFLD.[69] However, none of them are yet approved. Finally, it has been noted that glucagon-like peptide-1 receptor agonists can improve liver steatosis in patients with T2DM, and they may also increase lean mass via activation of GH/IGF-1 axis (**Table 1**).[70]

SUMMARY

Sarcopenia and MAFLD display an increasing prevalence in the modern world. Various pathophysiologic pathways can explain their coexistence, which is associated with worse clinical outcomes and mortality. Therefore, evaluation and quantification of sarcopenia may be of value in patients diagnosed with MAFLD. The current therapeutic recommendations for both diseases focus on lifestyle interventions, such as a balanced diet and daily exercise, even though new possible pharmacotherapeutic targets have been enlightened. Nevertheless, further studies are needed in order to develop updated guidelines for early detection and appropriate treatment but also for better comprehension of muscle-liver interactions, which will aid in development of precision medicine for optimal treatment.

CLINICS CARE POINTS

- Screening for sarcopenia in patients with MAFLD and vice versa may be of high value for optimal care in both conditions.
- Awareness of the need to optimize diet and physical activity, given the absence of approved drugs, is essential in patients with MAFLD and/or sarcopenia.

CONFLICT-OF-INTEREST

No potential conflicts of interest. No financial support.

REFERENCES

1. Zambon Azevedo V, Silaghi CA, Maurel T, et al. Impact of sarcopenia on the severity of the liver damage in patients with non-alcoholic fatty liver disease. Front Nutr 2021;8:774030.

2. Kuchay MS, Martinez-Montoro JI, Kaur P, et al. Non-alcoholic fatty liver disease-related fibrosis and sarcopenia: an altered liver-muscle crosstalk leading to increased mortality risk. Ageing Res Rev 2022;80:101696.

3. Fernandez-Mincone T, Contreras-Briceno F, Espinosa-Ramirez M, et al. Nonalcoholic fatty liver disease and sarcopenia: pathophysiological connections and therapeutic implications. Expet Rev Gastroenterol Hepatol 2020;14(12):1141–57.

4. Korenblat KM, Fabbrini E, Mohammed BS, et al. Liver, muscle, and adipose tissue insulin action is directly related to intrahepatic triglyceride content in obese subjects. Gastroenterology 2008;134(5):1369–75.

5. Le MH, Yeo YH, Li X, et al. 2019 Global NAFLD prevalence: a systematic review and meta-analysis. Clin Gastroenterol Hepatol 2022;20(12):2809–2817 e28.

6. Morley JE, Anker SD, von Haehling S. Prevalence, incidence, and clinical impact of sarcopenia: facts, numbers, and epidemiology-update 2014. J Cachexia Sarcopenia Muscle 2014;5(4):253–9.

7. El Sherif O, Dhaliwal A, Newsome PN, et al. Sarcopenia in nonalcoholic fatty liver disease: new challenges for clinical practice. Expet Rev Gastroenterol Hepatol 2020;14(3):197–205.

8. Santos CML, Brito MD, de Castro P, et al. Metabolic-associated fatty liver disease is associated with low muscle mass and strength in patients with chronic hepatitis B. World J Hepatol 2022;14(8):1652–66.

9. Petta S, Ciminnisi S, Di Marco V, et al. Sarcopenia is associated with severe liver fibrosis in patients with non-alcoholic fatty liver disease. Aliment Pharmacol Ther 2017;45(4):510–8.

10. Koo BK, Kim D, Joo SK, et al. Sarcopenia is an independent risk factor for non-alcoholic steatohepatitis and significant fibrosis. J Hepatol 2017;66(1):123–31.

11. Kim G, Lee SE, Lee YB, et al. Relationship between relative skeletal muscle mass and nonalcoholic fatty liver disease: a 7-year longitudinal study. Hepatology 2018;68(5):1755–68.

12. Lee YH, Jung KS, Kim SU, et al. Sarcopaenia is associated with NAFLD independently of obesity and insulin resistance: nationwide surveys (KNHANES 2008-2011). J Hepatol 2015;63(2):486–93.

13. Sun X, Liu Z, Chen F, et al. Sarcopenia modifies the associations of nonalcoholic fatty liver disease with all-cause and cardiovascular mortality among older adults. Sci Rep 2021;11(1):15647.

14. Kouvari M, Polyzos SA, Chrysohoou C, et al. Skeletal muscle mass and abdominal obesity are independent predictors of hepatic steatosis and interact to predict ten-year cardiovascular disease incidence: data from the ATTICA cohort study. Clin Nutr 2022;41(6):1281–9.

15. Papatheodoridi AM, Chrysavgis L, Koutsilieris M, et al. the role of senescence in the development of nonalcoholic fatty liver disease and progression to nonalcoholic steatohepatitis. Hepatology 2020;71(1):363–74.

16. Bertolotti M, Lonardo A, Mussi C, et al. Nonalcoholic fatty liver disease and aging: epidemiology to management. World J Gastroenterol 21 2014;20(39):14185–204.

17. Saad F, Röhrig G, von Haehling S, et al. Testosterone deficiency and testosterone treatment in older men. Gerontology 2017;63(2):144–56.

18. Lonardo A, Nascimbeni F, Ballestri S, et al. Sex differences in nonalcoholic fatty liver disease: state of the art and identification of research gaps. Hepatology 2019;70(4):1457–69.

19. Ford ES, Ajani UA, McGuire LC, et al. Concentrations of serum vitamin D and the metabolic syndrome among U.S. adults. Diabetes Care 2005;28(5):1228–30.

20. Velazquez KT, Enos RT, Bader JE, et al. Prolonged high-fat-diet feeding promotes non-alcoholic fatty liver disease and alters gut microbiota in mice. World J Hepatol 2019;11(8):619–37.

21. van den Hoek AM, de Jong J, Worms N, et al. Diet and exercise reduce pre-existing NASH and fibrosis and have additional beneficial effects on the vasculature, adipose tissue and skeletal muscle via organ-crosstalk. Metabolism 2021; 124:154873.

22. Mikolasevic I, Pavic T, Kanizaj TF, et al. Nonalcoholic fatty liver disease and sarcopenia: where do we stand? Chin J Gastroenterol Hepatol 2020;2020:8859719.

23. Longo M, Zatterale F, Naderi J, et al. Adipose tissue dysfunction as determinant of obesity-associated metabolic complications. Int J Mol Sci 2019;20(9):2358.

24. Kumar A, Welch N, Mishra S, et al. Metabolic reprogramming during hyperammonemia targets mitochondrial function and postmitotic senescence. JCI Insight 2021;6(24):e154089.

25. Kurose S, Onishi K, Takao N, et al. Association of serum adiponectin and myostatin levels with skeletal muscle in patients with obesity: a cross-sectional study. PLoS One 2021;16(1):e0245678.

26. Polyzos SA, Kountouras J, Anastasilakis AD, et al. Irisin in patients with nonalcoholic fatty liver disease. Metabolism 2014;63(2):207–17.

27. Powrozek T, Pigon-Zajac D, Mazurek M, et al. TNF-alpha induced myotube atrophy in C2C12 cell line uncovers putative inflammatory-related lncRNAs mediating muscle wasting. Int J Mol Sci 2022;23(7).

28. Cai D, Frantz JD, Tawa NE Jr, et al. IKKbeta/NF-kappaB activation causes severe muscle wasting in mice. Cell 2004;119(2):285–98.

29. Wong VW, Tse CH, Lam TT, et al. Molecular characterization of the fecal microbiota in patients with nonalcoholic steatohepatitis–a longitudinal study. PLoS One 2013;8(4):e62885.

30. Liu C, Cheung WH, Li J, et al. Understanding the gut microbiota and sarcopenia: a systematic review. J Cachexia Sarcopenia Muscle 2021;12(6):1393–407.

31. Hong SH, Choi KM. Sarcopenic obesity, insulin resistance, and their implications in cardiovascular and metabolic consequences. Int J Mol Sci 2020;21(2):494.

32. Stitt TN, Drujan D, Clarke BA, et al. The IGF-1/PI3K/Akt pathway prevents expression of muscle atrophy-induced ubiquitin ligases by inhibiting FOXO transcription factors. Mol Cell 2004;14(3):395–403.

33. Kim JA, Choi KM. Sarcopenia and fatty liver disease. Hepatol Int 2019;13(6): 674–87.

34. Cleasby ME, Jamieson PM, Atherton PJ. Insulin resistance and sarcopenia: mechanistic links between common co-morbidities. J Endocrinol 2016;229(2): R67–81.

35. Ji T, Li Y, Ma L. Sarcopenic obesity: an emerging public health problem. Aging Dis 2022;13(2):379–88.

36. Gao Q, Mei F, Shang Y, et al. Global prevalence of sarcopenic obesity in older adults: a systematic review and meta-analysis. Clin Nutr 2021;40(7):4633–41.

37. Song W, Yoo SH, Jang J, et al. Association between sarcopenic obesity status and nonalcoholic fatty liver disease and fibrosis. Gut Liver 2023;17(1):130–8.

38. Chun HS, Lee M, Lee HA, et al. Risk stratification for sarcopenic obesity in subjects with nonalcoholic fatty liver disease. Clin Gastroenterol Hepatol 2022. S1542-3565(22)01111-9.

39. Lim S, Kim JH, Yoon JW, et al. Sarcopenic obesity: prevalence and association with metabolic syndrome in the Korean Longitudinal Study on Health and Aging (KLoSHA). Diabetes Care 2010;33(7):1652–4.

40. Kim TN, Park MS, Kim YJ, et al. Association of low muscle mass and combined low muscle mass and visceral obesity with low cardiorespiratory fitness. PLoS One 2014;9(6):e100118.

41. Fielding RA, Vellas B, Evans WJ, et al. Sarcopenia: an undiagnosed condition in older adults. Current consensus definition: prevalence, etiology, and consequences. International working group on sarcopenia. J Am Med Dir Assoc 2011;12(4):249–56.

42. Welch AA, Hayhoe RPG, Cameron D. The relationships between sarcopenic skeletal muscle loss during ageing and macronutrient metabolism, obesity and onset of diabetes. Proc Nutr Soc 2020;79(1):158–69.

43. Polyzos SA, Margioris AN. Sarcopenic obesity. Hormones (Basel) 2018;17(3):321–31.

44. Cruz-Jentoft AJ, Bahat G, Bauer J, et al. Sarcopenia: revised European consensus on definition and diagnosis. Age Ageing 2019;48(1):16–31.

45. Malmstrom TK, Morley JE. SARC-F: a simple questionnaire to rapidly diagnose sarcopenia. J Am Med Dir Assoc 2013;14(8):531–2.

46. Donini LM, Busetto L, Bischoff SC, et al. Definition and diagnostic criteria for sarcopenic obesity: ESPEN and EASO consensus statement. Obes Facts 2022;15(3):321–35.

47. Merli M, Dasarathy S. Sarcopenia in non-alcoholic fatty liver disease: targeting the real culprit? J Hepatol 2015;63(2):309–11.

48. Aleixo GFP, Shachar SS, Nyrop KA, et al. Bioelectrical impedance analysis for the assessment of sarcopenia in patients with cancer: a systematic review. Oncol 2020;25(2):170–82.

49. Chianca V, Albano D, Messina C, et al. Sarcopenia: imaging assessment and clinical application. Abdom Radiol (NY) 2022;47(9):3205–16.

50. Giusto M, Lattanzi B, Albanese C, et al. Sarcopenia in liver cirrhosis: the role of computed tomography scan for the assessment of muscle mass compared with dual-energy X-ray absorptiometry and anthropometry. Eur J Gastroenterol Hepatol 2015;27(3):328–34.

51. Williams FR, Milliken D, Lai JC, et al. Assessment of the frail patient with end-stage liver disease: a practical overview of sarcopenia, physical function, and disability. Hepatol Commun 2021;5(6):923–37.

52. Dhaliwal A, Armstrong MJ. Sarcopenia in cirrhosis: a practical overview. Clin Med 2020;20(5):489–92.

53. Chrysavgis L, Giannakodimos I, Diamantopoulou P, et al. Non-alcoholic fatty liver disease and hepatocellular carcinoma: clinical challenges of an intriguing link. World J Gastroenterol 21 2022;28(3):310–31.

54. Zarghamravanbakhsh P, Frenkel M, Poretsky L. Metabolic causes and consequences of nonalcoholic fatty liver disease (NAFLD). Metabol Open 2021;12:100149.

55. Byrne CD, Targher G. NAFLD: a multisystem disease. J Hepatol 2015;62(1 Suppl):S47–64.

56. Targher G, Byrne CD, Lonardo A, et al. Non-alcoholic fatty liver disease and risk of incident cardiovascular disease: a meta-analysis. J Hepatol 2016;65(3):589–600.

57. AlQudah M, Hale TM, Czubryt MP. Targeting the renin-angiotensin-aldosterone system in fibrosis. Matrix Biol 2020;91-92:92–108.

58. Kim D, Wijarnpreecha K, Sandhu KK, et al. Sarcopenia in nonalcoholic fatty liver disease and all-cause and cause-specific mortality in the United States. Liver Int 2021;41(8):1832–40.

59. Bartekova M, Radosinska J, Jelemensky M, et al. Role of cytokines and inflammation in heart function during health and disease. Heart Fail Rev 2018;23(5): 733–58.
60. Moon JH, Koo BK, Kim W. Non-alcoholic fatty liver disease and sarcopenia additively increase mortality: a Korean nationwide survey. J Cachexia Sarcopenia Muscle 2021;12(4):964–72.
61. Han E, Kim MK, Im SS, et al. Non-alcoholic fatty liver disease and sarcopenia is associated with the risk of albuminuria independent of insulin resistance, and obesity. J Diabet Complications 2022;36(8):108253.
62. European Association for the Study of the L, European Association for the Study of D, European Association for the Study of O. EASL-EASD-EASO clinical practice guidelines for the management of non-alcoholic fatty liver disease. J Hepatol 2016;64(6):1388–402.
63. Richter EA, Hargreaves M. Exercise, GLUT4, and skeletal muscle glucose uptake. Physiol Rev 2013;93(3):993–1017.
64. Fredrickson G, Barrow F, Dietsche K, et al. Exercise of high intensity ameliorates hepatic inflammation and the progression of NASH. Mol Metab 2021;53:101270.
65. Zhang C, Yang M. Current options and future directions for NAFLD and NASH treatment. Int J Mol Sci 2021;22(14):7571.
66. Vancells Lujan P, Viñas Esmel E, Sacanella Meseguer E. Overview of non-alcoholic fatty liver disease (NAFLD) and the role of sugary food consumption and other dietary components in its development. Nutrients 2021;13(5):1442.
67. Sinclair M, Grossmann M, Hoermann R, et al. Testosterone therapy increases muscle mass in men with cirrhosis and low testosterone: a randomised controlled trial. J Hepatol 2016;65(5):906–13.
68. Mansour-Ghanaei F, Pourmasoumi M, Hadi A, et al. The efficacy of Vitamin D supplementation against nonalcoholic fatty liver disease: a meta-analysis. J Diet Suppl 2020;17(4):467–85.
69. Late breaker posters. J Hepatol 2021;75:S294–803.
70. Cignarelli A, Genchi VA, Le Grazie G, et al. Mini review: effect of GLP-1 receptor agonists and SGLT-2 Inhibitors on the growth hormone/IGF axis. Front Endocrinol 2022;13:846903.

A Bidirectional Association Between Obstructive Sleep Apnea and Metabolic-Associated Fatty Liver Disease

Anish Preshy, MBBS, MPHTM[a],*, James Brown, FRCP(Edin), FRACP[b]

KEYWORDS

- Metabolic-associated fatty liver disease • Obstructive sleep apnea
- Chronic intermittent hypoxia • Insulin resistance • Steatosis • Fibrosis • CPAP

KEY POINTS

- There is a strong association between metabolic-associated fatty liver disease (MAFLD) and obstructive sleep apnea (OSA).
- OSA is associated with a twofold increased risk of steatosis, steatohepatitis, and fibrosis, independent of obesity.
- OSA-induced insulin resistance, oxidative stress, gut dysbiosis, and molecular changes are all considered to contribute to the pathogenesis of MAFLD.

INTRODUCTION

Obstructive sleep apnea (OSA) is the most common type of sleep-disordered breathing.[1] OSA is characterized by ventilatory disruptions from repetitive upper respiratory airway collapse during sleep. This triggers periodic apnea, hypopneas, intra-thoracic pressure changes, derangements of gas exchange, sleep fragmentations, and repetitive intermittent hypoxia sequence (i.e., chronic intermittent hypoxia [CIH]).[2]

The presence of hepatic steatosis and signs of metabolic dysfunction, obesity, or diabetes defines metabolic-associated fatty liver disease (MAFLD).[3] In time, a certain proportion of patients develop inflammatory infiltration and hepatocyte ballooning, progressing to steatohepatitis and eventually progressing to liver cell injury and fibrosis. Emerging research indicates that MAFLD is a multi-system disease. The mechanism by which MAFLD progresses into non-alcoholic steatohepatitis (NASH)

[a] Department of Medicine, Cairns Hospital, Cairns, Queensland, Australia; [b] Department of Thoracic Medicine, Cairns Hospital, Cairns, Queensland, Australia
* Corresponding author. Department of Medicine, Cairns Hospital, 165 The Esplanade, Cairns, Queensland 4870, Australia
E-mail address: anish.preshy@health.qld.gov.au

Endocrinol Metab Clin N Am 52 (2023) 509–520
https://doi.org/10.1016/j.ecl.2023.01.006
0889-8529/23/© 2023 Elsevier Inc. All rights reserved.

is not entirely understood. Multiple mechanisms causing lipotoxicity, inflammation, and fibrosis have been postulated.

Although multiple pieces of literature explore the relationship between OSA and MAFLD, a complied literature review is lacking. This comprehensive review aims to compile, interlink, and delineate the available evidence to understand the pathophysiological, diagnostic, and management aspects of patients with OSA and MAFLD.

EPIDEMIOLOGY

Prevalence data from 17 epidemiological studies report that approximately 21% of the global population is estimated to have OSA.[4] The OSA prevalence increases with obesity, older age, male sex, and upper airway abnormalities.[4] OSA is associated with various metabolic complications, such as type 2 diabetes mellitus (T2DM) and MAFLD.

MAFLD has become the most common cause of chronic liver disease globally in recent years, paralleling the obesity epidemic worldwide. Current trends suggest that MAFLD may be present in about one-third of the global population.[5] NASH is projected to be the leading indication for liver transplantation in the future.[6]

A recent individual data meta-analysis from France has demonstrated that the prevalence of steatosis in severe OSA patients is 85%, among which 26% have signs of liver fibrosis.[7] A meta-analysis by Musso and colleagues[8] has conferred a twofold increase in the risk of steatosis, steatohepatitis, and fibrosis in OSA patients, independent of obesity. An OSA–MAFLD association has also been noted in the pediatric population, where 44% of non-obese and 68% of obese children with OSA were observed to have MAFLD.[9]

DIAGNOSTIC APPROACH

The gold standard diagnostic test for OSA is the attended in-laboratory polysomnography to estimate the apnea-hypopnea index (AHI).[10] Testing is currently recommended for patients with excessive daytime sleepiness, fatigue, and unrested sleep and should be considered in individuals with snoring, nocturnal awakenings, and gastroesophageal reflux.[11] The classification of OSA severity is based on the AHI; an AHI of 5 to 15 events per hour of sleep is classified as mild OSA, 15 to 30 events per hour as moderate, and $\geq$ 30 events per hour as severe.[12]

New guidelines for diagnosing MAFLD are based on radiological, histological, or non-invasive biomarkers for steatosis coupled with one or more of the following: (1) raised body mass index, (2) T2DM, or (3) two or more signs of metabolic risk abnormalities, including hypertension, increased glucose levels, insulin resistance (IR), high c-reactive protein, elevated waist circumference, and dyslipidemia.[3] The gold standard for MAFLD diagnosis remains to be a liver biopsy. However, given the invasive nature of a biopsy, ultrasound is recommended as the first-line test for detecting steatosis.[3] Ultrasound and vibration-controlled elastography are widely used in clinical practice, with computerised tomography (CT) or magnetic resonance imaging (MRI) being used to diagnose moderate to severe steatosis.[3] Upon confirming the diagnosis of MAFLD, the presence and extent of fibrosis can be detected using non-invasive biomarkers and liver stiffness markers. A definitive, reliable non-invasive scoring system is yet to be established.[13] However, a meta-analysis by Moze and colleagues[14] has established an algorithm sequentially combining non-invasive test cut-offs (Fibrosis-4 Index [FIB-4] and MAFLD fibrosis score [NFS]) with vibration-controlled transient elastography (fibroscan) to either rule out fibrosis or positively diagnose cirrhosis. Ideally, serum biomarkers combined with elastography could potentially replace the need for biopsy and imaging modalities in the future.

OBSTRUCTIVE SLEEP APNEA AND METABOLIC-ASSOCIATED FATTY LIVER DISEASE

Association Obesity on Obstructive Sleep Apnea and Metabolic-Associated Fatty Liver Disease

OSA leads to metabolic dysfunction via OSA-induced CIH and its downstream effects. These include sympathetic overactivity, oxidative stress, low-grade inflammation, dyslipidemia, and IR. Obesity and its consequent anatomical obstruction is a significant cause of sleep apnea.[15] The pathophysiology of OSA goes beyond the theory of anatomical obstruction. The physiological components of obesity, such as IR, elevated leptin levels, and glycemic control, can all contribute to the development of OSA.[16] Obesity may lead to sleep-disordered breathing and central sleep apnea through reduced respiratory mechano-receptor sensitivity via sympathetic overactivity and reduced pharyngeal muscle tone due to chronically increased muscle activity through inflammatory cascades (**Fig. 1**).[16]

A recent meta-analysis estimates the prevalence of obesity in MAFLD individuals at 50% and 80% for steatohepatitis.[17] In addition, prolonged exposure to CIH causing liver injury in diet-induced obese mice is similar to MAFLD in obese individuals with OSA.[18]

Risk of Metabolic-Associated Fatty Liver Disease in Obstructive Sleep Apnea

CIH and the repetitive desaturation and reoxygenation sequence is the most explored pathophysiological feature for the progression of metabolic dysfunction and subsequent MAFLD. The exact mechanism by which OSA causes hepato-metabolic alteration is unclear, but numerous studies (**Table 1**) support an association between MAFLD and OSA via both obesity-dependent and independent factors. There is emerging evidence in human studies affirming the degree of nocturnal hypoxemia in OSA being linked to the OSA–MAFLD association.[19]

Risk of Obstructive Sleep Apnea in Metabolic-Associated Fatty Liver Disease

There is a direct association between MAFLD and OSA. Recent studies suggest that MAFLD, defined by fatty liver index (FLI), independently increases the risk of OSA.[22,23] A US-based population study showed elevated liver enzyme-defined MAFLD was associated with sleep disorders.[24] The mechanism for this is unclear, and further randomized controlled trials (RCTs) are required to confirm the association. **Table 2** shows the studies showing MAFLD–OSA association.

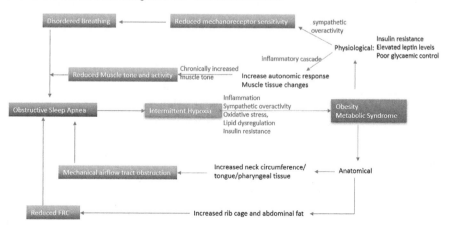

Fig. 1. OSA and obesity.

Table 1
Meta-analysis studies on obstructive sleep apnea–metabolic-associated fatty liver disease association

Study	Subjects (n)	Key Findings
Musso et al,[8] 2013	N = 2183	OSA is associated with a twofold increased risk of steatosis, steatohepatitis, and fibrosis, independent of obesity.
Jin et al,[20] 2018	N = 2272	OSA was significantly correlated with the development and progression of steatosis, ballooning degeneration, and fibrosis.
Jullian-Desayes et al,[7] 2020	N = 2120	There is a strong association between steatosis and OSA severity; 85% of severe OSA patients (AHI > 30 events/h) have steatosis. Risk factors for steatosis include AHI >5/h, male sex, higher age, excess body mass index (BMI), and diabetes.
Chen et al,[21] 2021	N = 1133	OSA was significantly associated with elevated liver transaminases and fibrosis in the pediatric population.

PATHOPHYSIOLOGY

No human studies have confirmed the tissue-specific effects of CIH. Multiple studies using experimental mice models show insight into the potential effects of CIH on the pathogenesis of MAFLD. Initially, a "two-hit" mechanism was hypothesized, where (1) hepatic lipid accumulation and IR followed by (2) inflammatory insults with oxidative stress resulting in steatohepatitis and fibrosis.[27] More recently, a "multi-parallel hit" process has been suggested, acting synergistically through various mechanisms.[27] CIH-induced IR and metabolic health, oxidative stress, gut dysbiosis, and molecular changes are all considered to contribute to the pathogenesis of MAFLD.

Chronic Intermittent Hypoxia, Insulin Resistance, and Metabolic Health

Multiple mechanisms are proposed by which CIH is an intermediate to IR, T2DM, and impaired glucose metabolism, independently of obesity (**Fig. 2**). CIH-induced systemic inflammation via nuclear factor kappa B (*NF-KB*) activation seems to be a key process in the pathogenesis of cardio-metabolic dysfunction. Activation of NF-KB leads to the

Table 2
Observational studies on metabolic-associated fatty liver disease-obstructive sleep apnea association

Study	Subjects (n)	Key Findings
Mir et al,[24] 2013 (population data)	N = 10,541	Individuals with MAFLD had a higher prevalence of sleep disorders.
Petta et al,[25] 2015	N = 126	OSA was highly prevalent in individuals with MAFLD, and severity was associated with the severity of liver fibrosis.
Cakmak et al,[26] 2015	N = 137	AHI and oxygen saturation indices were significantly higher in MAFLD compared to the non-MAFLD population.
Kim et al,[22] 2022 (population cohort)	N = 334,334	MAFLD is independently associated with OSA in the Korean population.
Chung et al,[23] 2021 (population cohort)	N = 8,116,524	The risk of OSA was significantly greater in patients with a higher FLI.

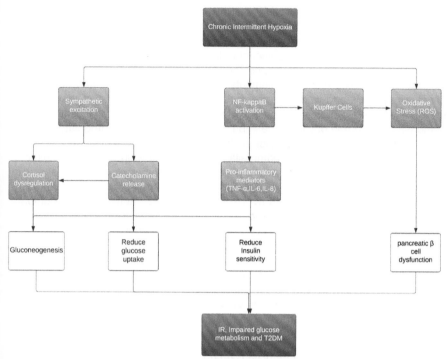

Fig. 2. *CIH and IR.* IL, interleukin; IR, insulin resistance; ROS, reactive oxidative species; T2DM, type 2 diabetes mellitus; TNF α, tumor necrosis factor-alpha.

production of numerous pro-inflammatory mediators.[28] Hypoxia and hypercapnia are found to stimulate the peripheral chemoreceptors triggering autonomic dysfunction and sympathetic hyperactivity.[29] There is an increased risk for liver steatosis secondary to CIH-induced sympathetic excitation and autonomic imbalance.[30] The underlying mechanisms postulated involve catecholamine and cortisol release secondary to sympathetic overactivity, resulting in reduced insulin sensitivity, glucose uptake, and increased gluconeogenesis.[28,31] Additionally, CIH is associated with increased production of reactive oxidative species (ROS) directly and indirectly through the activation of Kupffer cells and recruitment of activated phagocytes into the liver.[32,33]

Hypoxia induced by adipose tissue expansion also increases adipocyte dysfunction, proliferation, and subsequently lipolysis, leading to adipocyte inflammation, which results in an acute rise of plasma-free fatty acids (FFAs). Increased FFAs lead to lipid accumulation and gluconeogenesis, causing impaired insulin signaling and increased IR.[28] IR, via the various mechanisms mentioned above, leads to an increase of the sterol regulatory element-binding protein 1c (SREBP-1c) gene through (1) the downregulation of insulin receptor substrate 2 (IRS-2), (2) suppression of FFA β-oxidation, (3) the inhibition of lipolysis, and (4) stimulation of phosphatidylinositol-3 kinase (PI3K).[27,34] Increase of SREBP-1c results in de novo lipogenesis and, consequently, steatosis. Elevated insulin levels also directly stimulate PI3K resulting in apoptosis and inflammation of hepatocytes leading to steatohepatitis.[34]

Molecular Consequence of Chronic Intermittent Hypoxia

Previous studies have explored the role of activation of hypoxia-inducible factors (HIFs). These induce lipid accumulation in hepatocytes resulting in the development of MAFLD and further progression to steatohepatitis and fibrosis.[35] The cellular mechanisms of the human body are highly dependent on oxygen. Even a mild reduction in oxygen initiates a rapid adaptive oxygen response, after which activation of both the HIF and NF-KB pathways are significant to the development of MAFLD.[32] Sleep fragmentation/CIH exposure upregulates the expression of HIF1α complexes, which interact with hypoxic response elements to induce target genes with downstream effects on glucose and lipid metabolism, angiogenesis, and epithelial-mesenchymal transition, thereby, activating pro-inflammatory cascades.[32,35] Recent research demonstrated the role of CIH in the imbalance of Treg/Th17 cells (regulatory T cell/T helper cell 17) through the expression of the HIF1α subunit and subsequent activation of the mTOR-HIF1α-TLR4-IL-6 (mammalian target of rapamycin-HIF1α-toll-like receptor 4-interleukin-6) inflammatory pathway.[36] This exacerbates oxidative stress and induces hypoxia, accelerating the progression of steatohepatitis and liver fibrosis.

There is growing evidence that hypoxia-induced HIF2α activation, in addition to HIF1α activation, leads to the upregulation of genes involved in FFA uptake and hepatocyte lipid accumulation while suppressing lipid synthesis and β-oxidation.[37] An increase of HIF2α in hypoxic HepG2 cells also was shown to increase adipose differentiation-related protein expression, which results in further FFA uptake and steatosis.[38] An upregulation of HIF2α can also activate the NF-KB pathway and exacerbate steatohepatitis.[39] HIF2α may be a potential therapeutic target, given its implied role in the progression of steatosis to severe steatohepatitis and fibrosis.

Chronic Intermittent Hypoxia-Induced Oxidative Stress and Chronic Inflammation

Previous studies have demonstrated that prolonged exposure to CIH induces increased lipid peroxidation, independently of obesity.[40] Under hypoxic conditions, NF-KB activates Kupffer cells and generates ROS. An increase in ROS interacts with FFAs to induce lipid peroxidation and causes mitochondrial dysfunction and subsequent liver damage.[41] Recurrent sleep fragmentation and arousals may also incite endothelial dysfunction and increased inflammatory cytokine recruitment (such as interleukin (IL)-6).[42] In addition, Kupffer cells release inflammatory cytokines [IL-6, tumor necrosis factor-alpha (TNF-a)], which have been suggested to promote the development of MAFLD and progression into NASH.[32] A recent study on a mouse model explored the effect of CIH on MAFLD development and progression via the nuclear factor erythroid 2–related factor 2 (Nrf2)/NF-KB signaling pathway, modulated by the receptor-interacting serine/threonine-protein kinase 3 (RIPK3)-dependent necroptosis.[43] When RIPK3 is downregulated, hepatocyte necroptosis and subsequent inflammation and oxidative stress are ameliorated.[43] This opens new doors to exploring therapeutic strategies in OSA-induced MAFLD.

Chronic Intermittent Hypoxia and Alterations in Gut Microbiota

The association between OSA-induced alterations in gut microbiota and its effect on the liver has been explored in the pediatric population. In a mouse model, Nobili and colleagues[44] and Barcelo and colleagues[45] have suggested that OSA is associated with impaired gut permeability and intestinal damage resulting in elevated levels of lipopolysaccharide and endotoxins. This leads to low-grade inflammation and hepatocyte injury via upregulation of the hepatocyte Toll-like receptor 4 (TLR4).[44,45] Thus, OSA-induced gut–liver axis impairment contributes to MAFLD progression.

MANAGEMENT ALGORITHM

A clear management guideline to mitigate liver injury and prevent the complications of OSA and MAFLD is lacking. The aim should be to optimize metabolic sequelae and cardiovascular risk with early screening to prevent long-term complications of OSA and MAFLD. The cornerstone therapies for OSA and MAFLD continue to be behavioural and lifestyle modifications.

Behavioral/lifestyle changes

Multiple studies have shown good results in improving MAFLD and OSA with weight loss through exercise and diet control. Vilare-Gomez et al have demonstrated significant improvement in steatohepatitis in 90% of individuals with 7% to 10% weight loss (BW), with similar studies in Asia supporting this evidence.[46,47] Similarly, OSA patients with >10 kg weight loss have been shown to have a greater reduction in AHI of at least nine events/hour.[48] Exercise, independent of weight loss and diet, is also associated with a 20% reduction in OSA severity and intrahepatic triglycerides, hepatic steatosis, and liver stiffness.[49,50] Achieving and maintaining weight loss is challenging; hence an individualized, multi-disciplinary approach is required to assist and ensure motivation and continued participation.

Pharmacological management

There are multiple anti-diabetic medications reported to reduce weight, improve AHI, and protect against MAFLD, including glucagon-like peptide-1 receptor agonists .[51] Previous RCTs have demonstrated that Liraglutide is well tolerated and effective in reducing AHI and improving liver enzymes.[52,53] Other pharmacological agents reported to benefit MAFLD and OSA are antioxidants, such as vitamin E. However, evidence is lacking in MAFLD.[54] There are no FDA-approved drugs for MAFLD at this stage, but a few drugs (obeticholic acid, elafibranor, and selonsertib) have progressed to phase 3 development, showing evidence in reducing hepatic inflammation and fibrosis.[55] There are also emerging studies into novel therapeutic strategies targeting hypoxia and HIF factors.[56]

Continuous Positive Airway Pressure

Continuous positive airway pressure (CPAP) remains the gold standard therapy for OSA. Although the associations between OSA and MAFLD have been proven, large-scale RCTs on CPAP use in OSA and MAFLD have yet to demonstrate significant benefits on glucose levels, IR, or inflammatory markers, except in the improvement of blood pressure.[57–60] This questions a true association between the two conditions. The lack of evidence may be due to limited CPAP trials, poor CPAP compliance, or the multi-hit mode of MAFLD pathogenesis, in which CPAP only targets the CIH. Without targeting the other factors (among which especially obesity), a positive impact of CPAP on liver function may be challenging to establish. Furthermore, data on CPAP studies are predominately short-term. A more extended observational period in studies will be required to show the true effect of CPAP on MAFLD.

Metabolic/Bariatric Surgery

Among individuals who underwent bariatric surgery, MAFLD is present in the majority of patients (>90%) and OSA in 71% of patients.[61,62] Multiple studies have explored the effect of bariatric surgery on OSA and MAFLD, showing a resolution of steatosis in >75% of patients, and even suggesting a regression in fibrosis.[62] A meta-analysis on the effects of bariatric surgery on OSA reported that over 75% of patients had improved OSA outcomes and demonstrated more significant improvement in AHI than non-surgical interventions.[63] Bariatric surgery is considered the most efficacious management for obesity, although current guidelines still consider it premature to be offered as a first-line therapy.[64] This may be due to the lack of RCTs comparing bariatric surgery to other interventions (such as CPAP), making it difficult to assess the benefit and harm. However, in light of the evidence above, bariatric surgery should be considered for obese patients (BMI >35) with MAFLD and severe OSA.

CLINICS CARE POINTS

- The degree of OSA is linked to the MAFLD severity (A1)
- Patients with moderate to severe OSA should be routinely screened for MAFLD, with/without obesity (A2)
- Patients with MAFLD should be considered for OSA screening (B2)
- Sequentially combining non-invasive test cut-offs (FIB-4 and NFS) with vibration-controlled transient elastography (fibroscan) can rule out fibrosis and rule in cirrhosis (A2)
- Behavioral and lifestyle changes toward a healthy diet and exercise should be recommended in obese and non-obese individuals with MAFLD and OSA (B2)
- Weight loss of approximately 10% should be the target for improvement of OSA and MAFLD (B1)
- Liraglutide is well tolerated and is effective in reducing AHI and improving liver function tests (B1)
- CPAP alone does not provide any significant benefit in MAFLD (A2)
- Bariatric surgery should be considered for obese patients (BMI >35) with MAFLD and severe OSA (B1)

SUMMARY

In conclusion, the exact mechanisms for OSA causing MAFLD and vice versa are unclear, despite the well-established association between OSA and MAFLD. Previous research studies have shown a direct relationship between the severity of OSA and the degree of MAFLD. There is also a relationship between nocturnal hypoxemia and MAFLD severity. This may be due to the CIH burden of OSA. We can confirm that CIH-induced sympathetic overactivity, oxidative stress, low-grade inflammation, dyslipidemia, and IR are involved, but more in-depth studies are required to clarify the causal relationship between these factors and MAFLD. Additional long-term CPAP studies need to be designed and be more reflective of clinical practice to evaluate the liver's response to OSA treatment. A multimodal management plan is required as combined therapies, including weight loss and exercise in combination with pharmacological and CPAP management, have been shown to improve IR and triglyceride levels, influencing MAFLD and OSA outcomes.

DISCLOSURE

All authors have nil commercial or financial conflicts of interest.

ACKNOWLEDGMENTS

Nil.

REFERENCES

1. Lyons MM, Bhatt NY, Pack AI, et al. Global burden of sleep-disordered breathing and its implications. Respirology 2020;25(7):690–702.
2. Pengo MF, Bonafini S, Fava C, et al. Cardiorespiratory interaction with continuous positive airway pressure. J Thorac Dis 2018;10(Suppl 1):S57–70.
3. Eslam M, Newsome PN, Sarin SK, et al. A new definition for metabolic dysfunction-associated fatty liver disease: an international expert consensus statement. J Hepatol 2020;73(1):202–9.
4. Benjafield AV, Ayas NT, Eastwood PR, et al. Estimation of the global prevalence and burden of obstructive sleep apnoea: a literature-based analysis. Lancet Respir Med 2019;7(8):687–98.
5. Le MH, Yeo YH, Li X, et al. 2019 Global NAFLD prevalence: a systematic review and meta-analysis, Clin Gastroenterol Hepatol, 20, 12, 2022, 2809-2817.e28.
6. Wong RJ, Aguilar M, Cheung R, et al. Nonalcoholic steatohepatitis is the second leading etiology of liver disease among adults awaiting liver transplantation in the United States. Gastroenterology 2015;148(3):547–55.
7. Jullian-Desayes I, Trzepizur W, Boursier J, et al. Obstructive sleep apnea, chronic obstructive pulmonary disease and NAFLD: an individual participant data meta-analysis. Sleep Med 2021;77:357–64.
8. Musso G, Cassader M, Olivetti C, et al. Association of obstructive sleep apnoea with the presence and severity of non-alcoholic fatty liver disease. A systematic review and meta-analysis. Obes Rev 2013;14(5):417–31.
9. Isaza SC, Del Pozo-Maroto E, Domínguez-Alcón L, et al. Hypoxia and Non-alcoholic Fatty Liver Disease. Front Med 2020;7:578001.
10. Kapur VK, Auckley DH, Chowdhuri S, et al. Clinical practice guideline for diagnostic testing for adult obstructive sleep apnea: an american academy of sleep medicine clinical practice guideline. J Clin Sleep Med 2017;13(03):479–504.
11. Gottlieb DJ, Punjabi NM. Diagnosis and management of obstructive sleep apnea: a review. JAMA 2020;323(14):1389–400.
12. Douglas JA, Chai-Coetzer CL, McEvoy D, et al. Guidelines for sleep studies in adults - a position statement of the Australasian Sleep Association. Sleep Med 2017;36(Suppl 1):S2–22.
13. Wu YL, Kumar R, Wang MF, et al. Validation of conventional non-invasive fibrosis scoring systems in patients with metabolic-associated fatty liver disease. World J Gastroenterol 2021;27(34):5753–63.
14. Mózes FE, Lee JA, Selvaraj EA, et al. Diagnostic accuracy of non-invasive tests for advanced fibrosis in patients with NAFLD: an individual patient data meta-analysis. Gut 2022;71(5):1006–19.
15. Ryan CM, Bradley TD. Pathogenesis of obstructive sleep apnea. J Appl Physiol 2005;99(6):2440–50.
16. Framnes SN, Arble DM. The bidirectional relationship between obstructive sleep apnea and metabolic disease. Front Endocrinol 2018;9:440.
17. Younossi ZM, Koenig AB, Abdelatif D, et al. Global epidemiology of nonalcoholic fatty liver disease-Meta-analytic assessment of prevalence, incidence, and outcomes. Hepatology 2016;64(1):73–84.
18. Drager LF, Li J, Reinke C, et al. Intermittent hypoxia exacerbates metabolic effects of diet-induced obesity. Obesity 2011;19(11):2167–74.
19. Mesarwi OA, Loomba R, Malhotra A. Obstructive sleep apnea, hypoxia, and nonalcoholic fatty liver disease. Am J Respir Crit Care Med 2019;199(7):830–41.

20. Jin S, Jiang S, Hu A. Association between obstructive sleep apnea and non-alcoholic fatty liver disease: a systematic review and meta-analysis. Sleep Breath 2018;22(3):841–51.

21. Chen LD, Chen MX, Chen GP, et al. Association between obstructive sleep apnea and non-alcoholic fatty liver disease in pediatric patients: a meta-analysis. Pediatr Obes 2021;16(3):e12718.

22. Kim N, Roh J-H, Lee H, et al. The impact of non-alcoholic fatty liver disease on sleep apnea in healthy adults: A nationwide study of Korea. PLoS One 2022; 17(7):e0271021.

23. Chung GE, Cho EJ, Yoo J-J, et al. Nonalcoholic fatty liver disease is associated with the development of obstructive sleep apnea. Sci Rep 2021;11(1):13473.

24. Mir HM, Stepanova M, Afendy H, et al. Association of sleep disorders with nonalcoholic fatty liver disease (NAFLD): a population-based study. J Clin Exp Hepatol 2013;3(3):181–5.

25. Petta S, Marrone O, Torres D, et al. Obstructive sleep apnea is associated with liver damage and atherosclerosis in patients with non-alcoholic fatty liver disease. PLoS One 2015;10(12):e0142210.

26. Cakmak E, Duksal F, Altinkaya E, et al. Association between the severity of nocturnal hypoxia in obstructive sleep apnea and non-alcoholic fatty liver damage. Hepat Mon 2015;15(11):e32655.

27. Buzzetti E, Pinzani M, Tsochatzis EA. The multiple-hit pathogenesis of non-alcoholic fatty liver disease (NAFLD). Metabolism 2016;65(8):1038–48.

28. Ryan S. Adipose tissue inflammation by intermittent hypoxia: mechanistic link between obstructive sleep apnoea and metabolic dysfunction: Adipose tissue inflammation by intermittent hypoxia. J Physiol 2017;595(8):2423–30.

29. Iturriaga R, Alcayaga J, Chapleau MW, et al. Carotid body chemoreceptors: physiology, pathology, and implications for health and disease. Physiol Rev 2021;101(3):1177–235.

30. Jung I, Lee DY, Lee MY, et al. Autonomic imbalance increases the risk for non-alcoholic fatty liver disease. Front Endocrinol 2021;12:752944.

31. Kritikou I, Basta M, Vgontzas AN, et al. Sleep apnoea and the hypothalamic–pituitary–adrenal axis in men and women: effects of continuous positive airway pressure. Eur Respir J 2016;47(2):531–40.

32. Cai J, Hu M, Chen Z, et al. The roles and mechanisms of hypoxia in liver fibrosis. J Transl Med 2021;19(1):186.

33. Jaeschke H. Reactive oxygen and mechanisms of inflammatory liver injury: Present concepts. J Gastroenterol Hepatol 2011;26(s1):173–9.

34. Pal SC, Eslam M, Mendez-Sanchez N. Detangling the interrelations between MAFLD, insulin resistance, and key hormones. Hormones (Basel) Dec 2022; 21(4):573–89.

35. Lefere S, Van Steenkiste C, Verhelst X, et al. Hypoxia-regulated mechanisms in the pathogenesis of obesity and non-alcoholic fatty liver disease. Cell Mol Life Sci 2016;73(18):3419–31.

36. Liu J, Li W, Zhu W, et al. Chronic intermittent hypoxia promotes the development of experimental non-alcoholic steatohepatitis by modulating Treg/Th17 differentiation. Acta Biochim Biophys Sin 2018;50(12):1200–10.

37. Rankin EB, Rha J, Selak MA, et al. Hypoxia-inducible factor 2 regulates hepatic lipid metabolism. Mol Cell Biol 2009;29(16):4527–38.

38. Cao R, Zhao X, Li S, et al. Hypoxia Induces Dysregulation of Lipid Metabolism in HepG2 Cells via Activation of HIF-2α. Cell Physiol Biochem 2014;34(5):1427–41.

39. Cai H, Bai Z, Ge R-L. Hypoxia-inducible factor-2 promotes liver fibrosis in non-alcoholic steatohepatitis liver disease via the NF-κB signalling pathway. Biochem Biophys Res Commun 2021;540:67–74.

40. Savransky V, Nanayakkara A, Vivero A, et al. Chronic intermittent hypoxia predisposes to liver injury. Hepatology 2007;45(4):1007–13.

41. Wang J, Leclercq I, Brymora JM, et al. Kupffer cells mediate leptin-induced liver fibrosis. Gastroenterology 2009;137(2):713–23.

42. Carreras A, Zhang SX, Peris E, et al. Chronic sleep fragmentation induces endothelial dysfunction and structural vascular changes in mice. Sleep 2014;37(11):1817–24.

43. Zhang H, Zhou L, Zhou Y, et al. Intermittent hypoxia aggravates non-alcoholic fatty liver disease via RIPK3-dependent necroptosis-modulated Nrf2/NFκB signaling pathway. Life Sci 2021;285:119963.

44. Nobili V, Alisi A, Cutrera R, et al. Altered gut–liver axis and hepatic adiponectin expression in OSAS: novel mediators of liver injury in paediatric non-alcoholic fatty liver. Thorax 2015;70(8):769–81.

45. Barceló A, Esquinas C, Robles J, et al. Gut epithelial barrier markers in patients with obstructive sleep apnea. Sleep Med 2016;26:12–5.

46. Vilar-Gomez E, Martinez-Perez Y, Calzadilla-Bertot L, et al. Weight Loss Through Lifestyle Modification Significantly Reduces Features of Nonalcoholic Steatohepatitis. Gastroenterology 2015;149(2):367–78.e5.

47. Wong VW-S, Chan RS-M, Wong GL-H, et al. Community-based lifestyle modification programme for non-alcoholic fatty liver disease: a randomized controlled trial. J Hepatol 2013;59(3):536–42.

48. Foster GD, Borradaile KE, Sanders MH, et al. A randomized study on the effect of weight loss on obstructive sleep apnea among obese patients with type 2 diabetes: the Sleep AHEAD study. Arch Intern Med 2009;169(17):1619–26.

49. Orci LA, Gariani K, Oldani G, et al. Exercise-based interventions for nonalcoholic fatty liver disease: a meta-analysis and meta-regression. Clin Gastroenterol Hepatol 2016;14(10):1398–411.

50. Mendelson M, Lyons OD, Yadollahi A, et al. Effects of exercise training on sleep apnoea in patients with coronary artery disease: a randomised trial. Eur Respir J 2016;48(1):142–50.

51. Iqbal J, Wu HX, Hu N, et al. Effect of glucagon-like peptide-1 receptor agonists on body weight in adults with obesity without diabetes mellitus-a systematic review and meta-analysis of randomized control trials. Obes Rev 2022;23(6):e13435.

52. Khoo J, Hsiang J, Taneja R, et al. Comparative effects of liraglutide 3 mg vs structured lifestyle modification on body weight, liver fat and liver function in obese patients with non-alcoholic fatty liver disease: a pilot randomized trial. Diabetes Obes Metab 2017;19(12):1814–7.

53. Blackman A, Foster GD, Zammit G, et al. Effect of liraglutide 3.0 mg in individuals with obesity and moderate or severe obstructive sleep apnea: the SCALE Sleep Apnea randomized clinical trial. Int J Obes 2016;40(8):1310–9.

54. Lavine JE, Schwimmer JB, Van Natta ML, et al. Effect of vitamin E or metformin for treatment of nonalcoholic fatty liver disease in children and adolescents: the TONIC randomized controlled trial. JAMA 2011;305(16):1659–68.

55. Eslam M, Sarin SK, Wong VW, et al. The Asian Pacific Association for the Study of the Liver clinical practice guidelines for the diagnosis and management of metabolic-associated fatty liver disease. Hepatol Int 2020;14(6):889–919.

56. Foglia B, Novo E, Protopapa F, et al. Hypoxia, hypoxia-inducible factors and liver fibrosis, Cells, 10(7):2021;1764.
57. Ng SSS, Wong VWS, Wong GLH, et al. Continuous positive airway pressure does not improve nonalcoholic fatty liver disease in patients with obstructive sleep apnea. A randomized clinical trial. Am J Respir Crit Care Med 2021;203(4):493–501.
58. Labarca G, Cruz R, Jorquera J. Continuous positive airway pressure in patients with obstructive sleep apnea and non-alcoholic steatohepatitis: a systematic review and meta-analysis. J Clin Sleep Med 2018;14(1):133–9.
59. Peker Y, Balcan B. Cardiovascular outcomes of continuous positive airway pressure therapy for obstructive sleep apnea. J Thorac Dis 2018;10(Suppl 34): S4262–79.
60. Sharma SK, Agrawal S, Damodaran D, et al. CPAP for the metabolic syndrome in patients with obstructive sleep apnea. N Engl J Med 2011;365(24):2277–86.
61. Peromaa-Haavisto P, Tuomilehto H, Kössi J, et al. Prevalence of obstructive sleep apnoea among patients admitted for bariatric surgery. A prospective multicentre trial. Obes Surg 2016;26(7):1384–90.
62. Aguilar-Olivos NE, Almeda-Valdes P, Aguilar-Salinas CA, et al. The role of bariatric surgery in the management of nonalcoholic fatty liver disease and metabolic syndrome. Metab, Clin Exp 2015;65(8):1196–207.
63. Ashrafian H, Toma T, Rowland SP, et al. Bariatric surgery or non-surgical weight loss for obstructive sleep apnoea? A systematic review and comparison of meta-analyses. Obes Surg 2015;25(7):1239–50.
64. Chalasani N, Younossi Z, Lavine JE, et al. The diagnosis and management of nonalcoholic fatty liver disease: practice guidance from the American Association for the Study of Liver Diseases. Hepatology 2018;67(1):328–57.

Pregnancy and Metabolic-Associated Fatty Liver Disease

Claudia Mandato, PhD, MD[a], Nadia Panera, PhD[b], Anna Alisi, PhD[b],*

KEYWORDS

- Children - Metabolic-associated fatty liver disease - Nonalcoholic fatty liver disease
- Offspring - Pregnancy

KEY POINTS

- Because preexisting or de novo nonalcoholic fatty liver disease (NAFLD) during pregnancy may increase the risk of maternal and offspring complications, it is plausible that metabolic-associated fatty liver disease (MAFLD) may cause similar or more severe adverse outcomes.
- Only a few studies evaluated the nexus between maternal MAFLD and its effects on pregnant women and newborns.
- More prospective studies are needed to evaluate the adverse clinical outcomes associated with MAFLD in pregnancy.

INTRODUCTION

Although the debate on the new nomenclature is still open, the new definition of metabolic-associated fatty liver disease (MAFLD), even in children, seems to fully reproduce the pathophysiologic aspects of liver disease that characterize nonalcoholic fatty liver disease (NAFLD), but undoubtedly brings out the need to take into careful consideration the metabolic aspects that fill the constellation of comorbidities associated with NAFLD.[1] Indeed, the new definition of MAFLD comprises the diagnosis of fatty liver confirmed by liver histology, imaging, blood biomarkers, or blood scores combined with at least one of other conditions. These conditions include excess adiposity, prediabetes, or type 2 diabetes mellitus, and two metabolic abnormalities, such as increased waist circumference, hypertriglyceridemia, low levels of high-density lipoprotein cholesterol levels, impaired fasting glucose, and hypertension.[1]

[a] Department of Medicine, Surgery and Dentistry "Scuola Medica Salernitana", University of Salerno, Baronissi, Italy; [b] Genetics of Complex Phenotypes Research Unit, Bambino Gesù Children's Hospital, IRCCS, Viale S. Paolo, 15, Rome 00146, Italy
* Corresponding author.
E-mail address: anna.alisi@opbg.net

Endocrinol Metab Clin N Am 52 (2023) 521–531
https://doi.org/10.1016/j.ecl.2023.02.005   endo.theclinics.com

There is a scarcity of prospective epidemiologic studies after the new name (MAFLD) was adapted. However, a recent meta-analysis, which repurposes some existing epidemiologic data on fatty liver disease, found that the global prevalence of MAFLD is approximately 33% in the adult population, with varying distribution among the geographic areas.[2] Moreover, further meta-analyses estimated a MAFLD prevalence of 50.7% in the general population among overweight/obese adults, and of 44.94% in a special population based on data from pediatric obesity clinics.[3,4]

Recent retrospective studies in humans have investigated the prevalence of NAFLD during pregnancy highlighting that this condition may influence maternal and offspring outcomes, including gestational diabetes mellitus (GDM), gestational hypertension, caesarean delivery, preterm birth, preeclampsia, and abnormal fetal growth.[5-7] In particular, Sarkar and colleagues,[7] evaluating retrospectively data from a US database, reported that the prevalence of NAFLD in pregnancy increased in a timeframe of 9 years, with a rate of 10.5/100,000 pregnancies in 2007 and of 28.9/100,000 pregnancies in 2015. The authors also showed that metabolic comorbidities were more common in pregnant women with NAFLD where the risk of serious maternal and perinatal complications was significantly higher than in pregnant women with or without other chronic liver diseases. Similar results were confirmed in a study on 308,095 women registered in a Korean database, were NAFLD before pregnancy was strongly correlated with an increased risk of GDM.[8] Although all these clinical studies indicated that the adverse risks of obesity, metabolic syndrome, and NAFLD may affect maternal and perinatal outcomes, there are currently few lines of evidence whether the maternal MAFLD could be associated with more severe pregnancy-related complications in experimental mice models and humans.

In this review, we report all preclinical and clinical lines of evidence that may support the nexus between MAFLD and maternal and fetal outcomes during pregnancy, with an initial outline on the possible NAFLD murine models that may better recapitulate MAFLD.

PRECLINICAL MODELS FOR MATERNAL METABOLIC-ASSOCIATED FATTY LIVER DISEASE AND EFFECTS ON MATERNAL OUTCOMES DURING PREGNANCY

In the past, the development of a variety of dietary, genetic, chemical, and animal models of NAFLD have been established providing an invaluable tool for understanding the pathophysiologic mechanisms underlying the onset of NAFLD and its progression in terms of hepatic damage and metabolic dysregulation involving other organs.[9] These preclinical studies as described by Parthasarathy and colleagues,[10] have contributed to describe the so called "triadic lesion" concept that recapitulates the major hepatic features in NAFLD/nonalcoholic steatohepatitis (NASH), including hepatocyte injury, macrophage-mediated inflammation, and hepatic stellate cell activation, even if often the liver damage in animal models does not reach the severity observed in humans.

Currently, following the introduction of the new definition of NAFLD that shifts toward MAFLD, emphasis should be placed on the possibility to establish new models with an ability to fully mimic the systemic metabolic dysregulation and the hepatic injury occurring in the disease; or to use already available models for NAFLD/NASH, capable of reproducing the metabolic disorder emerging as dynamics-driven events into MAFLD. To date, there are no available models generated to resemble the MAFLD spectrum in humans, and most of the preclinical studies use animal models of NAFLD/NASH that also exhibit metabolic derangement.[11]

Table 1 summarizes the most suitable diet-induced obesity animal models (DIOs) for MAFLD and their characteristics.

Table 1
NAFLD models that recapitulate MAFLD

Type of DIOs Model	Type of Diet	Liver Damage	Dysmetabolic Phenotype
HFD	60% fat, 20% proteins, 20% carbohydrates	Complete spectrum of liver damage depending on time of diet regimen: steatosis in 10 wk and nonalcoholic steatohepatitis and fibrosis in >50 wk	Insulin resistance and hyperlipidemia in 10–12 wk
American lifestyle–induced obesity syndrome	45% calories in the chow from fat, 13% polyunsaturated fatty acids plus high-fructose corn syrup (55:45 wt/wt of fructose/glucose)	Complete spectrum of liver damage (hepatic steatosis, inflammation, and fibrosis) after 26 wk in mice	Obesity, metabolic syndrome, and dyslipidemia and insulin resistance after 16 wk in mice and 8 wk in rats
HFD and cholesterol	60% fat from cocoa butter and additional cholesterol (1.25% cholesterol and 0.5% cholate)	Complete spectrum of liver damage after 6–24 wk in mice	Oxidative stress and dyslipidemia, but not systemic insulin resistance

Abbreviations: DIO, diet-induced obesity; HFD, high-fat diet.

Among the animal models already established, those that best succeed in reproducing the full spectrum of hepatic and metabolic dysregulation occurring in MAFLD (eg, obesity, insulin resistance, and dyslipidemia) are those based on obesogenic DIO diets mainly developed in mice. The best studied DIO models are generally based on the administration of a regular high-fat diet (HFD). In particular, HFD with fat content up to 60% resulted usually in obesity and insulin resistance leading to a dysmetabolic phenotype after 10 to 12 weeks, including obesity, moderate hyperglycemia, hyperinsulinemia, and hypertriglyceridemia.[12] Mice fed an HFD develop a complete spectrum of liver damage, but it depends on the form and duration of the diet. Generally, they developed steatosis within 10 weeks, but it takes up to 36 weeks to develop hepatocyte ballooning and 52 weeks to NASH and fibrosis traits.[13]

However, several DIO models characterized by diets with different composition and types of sugars and fats have been established over time. Indeed, variations of the HFD composition with different type and ratio of carbohydrates and/or fat, such as additions of fructose or cholesterol in rodent DIOs, were found to be the most effective combination in mediating the more severe metabolic dysregulation and liver phenotype observed in humans.[13] According to a database of 3920 rodent models of NAFLD analyzed by a recent systematic review, the HFD/high-fructose diets were identified as the models that most closely resemble the human phenotype of NAFLD.[14] In fact, the American lifestyle–induced obesity syndrome diet composed of 45% calories (chow standard diet) from fat, 13% polyunsaturated fatty acids (PUFAs), with addition of high-fructose corn syrup (55:45 wt/wt of fructose/glucose) was found to affect metabolic systems in mice and rat models. More specifically, American lifestyle–induced obesity syndrome diet in mice was reported to promote obesity, metabolic syndrome, dyslipidemia, and insulin resistance after 16 weeks, and features of hepatic steatosis, inflammation, and fibrosis after 26 weeks. Similar metabolic dysfunction has been reported in rat models after only 8 weeks of treatment.[15]

The combination of HFD (60% fat from cocoa butter) and cholesterol supplementation (1.25% cholesterol and 0.5% cholate) was able to induce a more rapid and severe development of liver phenotype associated to NAFLD accompanied by metabolic disorders. After 6 to 24 weeks, steatosis, histologic NASH (inflammation, hepatocellular ballooning) features, and F1-F2 fibrosis were observed, whereas F3 fibrosis was appreciable only after 24 weeks.[16,17]

Experimental studies based on the previously described models highlighted that maternal overnutrition during pregnancy may lead to phenotypic changes in offspring, thus resembling human MAFLD.[18]

In most studies, the effect on the liver and on metabolic dysregulation were not investigated together. In mice during pregnancy, HFD may cause fatty liver and eventually liver fibrosis, changes in body composition, increased visceral adiposity, dyslipidemia, insulin resistance, reduced glucose tolerance related to reduced β-cell mass, and GDM.[18,19] A pattern of metabolic disorders more evident in mothers was instead observed in mouse models treated with a diet rich in fat and sucrose, where the NAFLD pattern could be associated with a state of low-grade systemic inflammation that may lead to MAFLD features.[18–20]

EFFECT OF METABOLIC-ASSOCIATED FATTY LIVER DISEASE ON MATERNAL OUTCOMES DURING PREGNANCY: CLINICAL EVIDENCE

NAFLD is nowadays considered as an independent risk factor for hypertensive complications, postpartum hemorrhage, and preterm birth. It is mandatory that NAFLD should be considered a high-risk obstetric condition, with clinical implications for counseling about potential obstetric complications and appropriate pregnancy care.[7]

The association between MAFLD and negative maternal outcomes during pregnancy was only recently reported in humans. Indeed, Lee and colleagues[21] have recently tried to define the risk of pregnancy complications according to the definitions of NAFLD and MAFLD by secondary analysis of a multicenter prospective cohort. The authors found that pregnant women with MAFLD exhibited the highest risk of adverse pregnancy outcomes including GDM, hypertension, and caesarean delivery compared with those with NAFLD without metabolic dysfunction. These results highlight that a preexisting maternal metabolic derangement may play a central role in the pathogenesis of adverse pregnancy outcomes, and that fatty liver may have an additive effect by triggering same or different pathways associated with these adverse outcomes. Systemic inflammation driven by obesity, insulin resistance, and NAFLD could be the detrimental mechanism that leads to adverse outcomes in pregnant women, such as preeclampsia.[22]

An inverse association of prolonged breastfeeding with the prevalence of NAFLD and metabolic alterations in middle age including body mass index (BMI), insulin resistance, elevated triglyceride levels, and waist circumference was also observed in women from the Coronary Artery Risk Development in Young Adults cohort.[23]

The mother's metabolic phenotype associated to a MAFLD pattern could be relevant in changes at the level of gut microbiota composition, which in turn may affect maternal insulin sensitivity and secretion during pregnancy.[24]

RESEARCH EVIDENCE ON THE EFFECTS OF MATERNAL METABOLIC-ASSOCIATED FATTY LIVER DISEASE ON OFFSPRING OUTCOMES

Because most of the obesogenic diets may affect offspring phenotype, several experimental models have described their effects including alterations in fetal growth, obesity, NAFLD, altered pancreatic β-cell mass, insulin resistance, and hypertension.[18]

Studies in several models, including those in mice, support the developmental programming of weight gain and metabolism in the offspring, demonstrating that obesogenic diets during pregnancy can transmit a propensity for adiposity, glucose intolerance, and cardiovascular dysfunction to the newborn.[25,26] However, most studies in mice were conducted by investigating the effect of maternal obesogenic diets before and during pregnancy and lactation on offspring weight gain, fatty liver, and dysmetabolism.[27,28]

A study investigating the effects of consumption of HFD in utero and during lactation reported excessive body weight, and the presence of fatty liver and insulin resistance in the offspring.[26] Moreover, Marin and colleagues[27] reported that in juvenile male mice fed with HFD plus fructose in the drinking water, the progression of liver damage and NASH development is faster than in juvenile female mice.

The role of maternal diet on offspring metabolic balance was well evaluated by de Paula Simino and colleagues.[28] The authors showed that in female mice on HFD, overnutrition during gestational and lactation periods disrupted lipid and glucose metabolism affecting glucose tolerance and insulin sensitivity in newborn by modifying the expression of hepatic miRNAs associated with insulin resistance and NAFLD. In addition, these changes increased the offspring susceptibility to obesity and metabolic derangement in adult life.

In female mice fed with a normal-fat diet or HFD for 12 weeks before conception and then during pregnancy and lactation, it was observed that appropriate dietary interventions initiated sufficiently early before pregnancy and continued also during lactation reduced the risk of offspring developing MAFLD even after the exposure to a maternal HFD.[29]

Animal experiments observed that maternal exposure to HFD during pregnancy and lactation could have lasting effects on increasing insulin resistance, associated with hepatic inflammation even in offspring with normal weight.[30]

There are several mechanisms that may link maternal DIO phenotype to offspring changes, including oxidative stress, epigenetic regulation of gene transcription, and changes in microbiota composition.[30–32] Indeed, maternal HFD caused metabolic dysfunction, including altered liver growth and oxidative stress thus contributing to NAFLD and the alteration of cholesterol levels in offspring.[30] Moreover, it has been reported that HFD consumption may induce epigenetic regulation of important genes involved in fatty acid oxidation and oxidative phosphorylation via DNA methylation modifications.[31] Wankhade and colleagues[32] demonstrated that even though HFD consumption in mice caused a strong alteration of the gut microbiome composition, the effects on weight gain, fatty liver, and metabolic dysfunction were dominant only in the male offspring.

A recent systematic review that investigated the metabolic repercussions of maternal exposure to HFD on offspring reported that exposures prepregnancy and during pregnancy and/or lactation was associated with increased body weight, food intake, and body adiposity in young and adult offspring.[33]

CLINICAL EVIDENCE ON THE EFFECT OF MATERNAL METABOLIC-ASSOCIATED FATTY LIVER DISEASE ON PROGENY

In addition to the evidence in mice models, a large number of clinical studies suggest that children born of pregnancies characterized by obesity or related GDM exhibited an increased risk of obesity, increased adiposity, impaired glucose tolerance, NAFLD, and other metabolic derangements.[34,35] Moreover, several studies highlighted how the mother's lifestyle and obesity during pregnancy can influence the short- and long-term metabolic pathways of the newborn child.[36] Hence, a clinical score has been proposed to calculate the risk of obesity based on the first thousand days of life.[37]

Cinelli and colleagues[38] evaluated the relationship between maternal and offspring (cord-blood) erythrocyte fatty acids at birth, in relation to prepregnancy BMI and gestational weight gain. The study showed that prepregnancy BMI but not gestational weight gain was correlated with changes in lipid profile in fetus including percentage of PUFAs, omega-6 fatty acid, and docosahexaenoic acid. The same authors demonstrated that the content of omega-3 PUFAs of maternal dietary intake during pregnancy influences the offspring DNA methylation profile, finding a correlation between erythrocytes membrane PUFA content and epigenetic regulation in offspring cord blood. In particular, it has been found that four genes (MSTN, IFNA13, ATP8B3, and GABBR2) mainly involved in the insulin resistance and adiposity development and phospholipid translocation across cell membranes were differentially methylated, among low, medium, and high omega-3 PUFA maternal intake groups.[39]

Furthermore, metagenomics studies have reported the possible maternal-fetal transmission of the intestinal microbiota, mainly characterized by Bifidobacterium and Bacteroides, during pregnancy and breastfeeding.[40] Infants receiving exclusive breast milk exhibited an increase in some taxa, such as Bifidobacterium and Lactobacillus spp, in respect to the formula-fed infants that showed high levels of Firmicutes.[41] This could be a reasonable explanation for the protective effect of breastfeeding on the subsequent development of NAFLD.[42] Breastfeeding also reduces the risk of MAFLD in mothers.[43]

GDM alone and together with maternal overweight/obesity impacts colonization of infant's gut influencing the amount of several taxa thus favoring a microbiome profile that could be associated with future risk of the metabolic dysregulation and MAFLD in childhood.[44–46] Moreover, children of obese women showed an increased risk to have MAFLD in adolescence.[34] This evidence was reinforced by a study demonstrating that children exposed in utero to maternal MAFLD may be more likely to exhibit early obesity and MAFLD.[47]

Unfortunately, the number of studies evaluating MAFLD and fetal outcomes is extremely small compared with those reported on NAFLD and extensively described by Fouda and colleagues.[6]

A study focused on the relationship between breastfeeding duration, breast milk composition, maternal obesity, and their effects on the rate of NAFLD during adolescence.[48] In particular, the study reported that high prepregnancy BMI correlates with less than 6 months of exclusive breastfeeding, which in turn is associated with a significantly increased risk of NAFLD in late adolescence and adverse metabolic profile. However, a similar study based on the Avon Longitudinal Study of Parents and Children (ALSPAC), while confirming the impact of maternal prepregnancy BMI on NAFLD development in the offspring, does not provide evidence regarding the protective role of exclusive breastfeeding greater than or equal to 6 months on NAFLD in young adulthood.[49] These last lines of evidence shed light on the relevance of lifestyle changes to prevent MAFLD in such children born to mothers with the disease.

MANAGEMENT OF METABOLIC-ASSOCIATED FATTY LIVER DISEASE IN PREGNANCY

The management of MAFLD in pregnancy includes early diagnosis, and a comprehensive medical support to carry out preventive measures and nutritional approaches that may reduce the risk of MAFLD-related adverse outcomes.[6] In these conditions, preconception counseling and an appropriate nutritional management during pregnancy are recommended.

Obese women with preexisting MAFLD should be monitored during pregnancy for high-risk obstetric complications, such as the exacerbation of already existing pathologies, hypertension, bleeding after delivery, and preterm birth.[6] Moreover, a baby who is born to a mother with MAFLD should be considered at risk of MAFLD during childhood. Breastfeeding and healthy weaning should be strongly promoted.[42,43] In these children, clinical and auxologic parameters must be closely monitored over time to suspect MAFLD early, possibly looking for biochemical abnormalities, such as reduced glucose tolerance, dyslipidemia, and alteration of liver function tests. Because there is no currently approved pharmacotherapy for MAFLD management in pregnancy, the treatment is mainly by lifestyle interventions, such as healthy diet and appropriate physical activities permitted during pregnancy.

SUMMARY AND FUTURE DIRECTIONS

MAFLD, the term proposed to substitute NAFLD, includes not only the hepatic manifestation of a multisystem disorder but also the associated metabolic dysfunction. There is currently inadequate clinical evidence showing that similar to NAFLD, maternal MAFLD can exist before pregnancy or can develop de novo during pregnancy thus influencing clinical outcomes in pregnant women and newborns. This limitation could be linked to the high heterogeneity that characterizes MAFLD, thus making the reproduction of laboratory evidence of systemic metabolic dysregulation and hepatic injury difficult in experimental models.

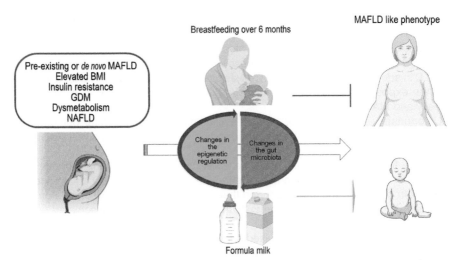

Fig. 1. Potential effects of preexisting or de novo maternal NAFLD and its associated metabolic dysregulation on MAFLD outcome in the pregnant woman and newborn. (Created with BioRender.com.)

However, based on the reported findings, metabolic adaptation caused by epigenetic remodeling of gene expression and/or microbiota composition could play a central role in pregnancy outcomes. Changes in epigenetic regulation that could be inherited, and alterations in the gut microbiome during fetal life may affect the metabolic response of the mother and child in animal models and humans (**Fig. 1**).[50] These metabolic changes are potentially reversible if unhealthy diet and adverse lifestyle are corrected during pregnancy, and by encouraging breastfeeding or the use of appropriate formula milk in the postpartum period.

CLINICS CARE POINTS

- MAFLD has emerged as a major health challenge in recent years because of the global obesity pandemic.

- Epigenetic, genetic, and environmental factors, such as adverse lifestyles, alterations in gut microbiome, and breastfeeding, may impact maternal and fetal outcomes in relation to MAFLD.

- Because there is no currently approved pharmacotherapy for MAFLD, and the difficulty in performing clinical trials among pregnant women, management of the disease during pregnancy is mainly by lifestyle interventions along with encouraging breastfeeding during the postpartum period.

- Obese women with dysmetabolism, GDM, or MAFLD should be monitored during pregnancy for high-risk obstetric conditions, such as the exacerbation of already existing pathologies, hypertension, bleeding after delivery, and preterm birth.

- A baby who is born to a mother with MAFLD should be screened as early as possible also for fatty liver by hepatic function tests and abdominal ultrasound.

- In these conditions, preconception counseling and accurate nutritional management during pregnancy can help avoid adverse maternal and offspring clinical outcomes.

DISCLOSURE

No conflict of interest.

FUNDING

This work was supported by the Italian Ministry of Health with "5x1000 2022".

REFERENCES

1. Eslam M, Alkhouri N, Vajro P, et al. Defining paediatric metabolic (dysfunction)-associated fatty liver disease: an international expert consensus statement. Lancet Gastroenterol Hepatol 2021;6:864–73.
2. Ayada I, van Kleef LA, Alferink LJM, et al. Systematically comparing epidemiological and clinical features of MAFLD and NAFLD by meta-analysis: focusing on the non-overlap groups. Liver Int 2022;42:277–87.
3. Liu J, Ayada I, Zhang X, et al. Estimating global prevalence of metabolic dysfunction-associated fatty liver disease in overweight or obese adults. Clin Gastroenterol Hepatol 2022;20:e573–82.
4. Liu J, Mu C, Li K, et al. Estimating global prevalence of metabolic dysfunction-associated fatty liver disease in overweight or obese children and adolescents: systematic review and meta-analysis. Int J Public Health 2021;66:1604371.
5. Mousa N, Abdel-Razik A, Shams M, et al. Impact of non-alcoholic fatty liver disease on pregnancy. Br J Biomed Sci 2018;75:197–9.
6. Fouda S, Vennikandam MM, Pappachan JM, et al. Pregnancy and metabolic-associated fatty liver disease: a clinical update. J Clin Transl Hepatol 2022;10: 947–54.
7. Sarkar M, Grab J, Dodge JL, et al. Non-alcoholic fatty liver disease in pregnancy is associated with adverse maternal and perinatal outcomes. J Hepatol 2020;73: 516–22.
8. You SY, Han K, Lee SH, et al. Nonalcoholic fatty liver disease and the risk of insulin-requiring gestational diabetes. Diabetol Metab Syndr 2021;13:90.
9. Gallage S, Avila JEB, Ramadori P, et al. A researcher's guide to preclinical mouse NASH models. Nat Metab 2022;4:1632–49.
10. Parthasarathy G, Revelo X, Malhi H. Pathogenesis of nonalcoholic steatohepatitis: an overview. Hepatol Commun 2020;4:478–92.
11. Chua D, Low ZS, Cheam GX, et al. Utility of human relevant preclinical animal models in navigating NAFLD to MAFLD paradigm. Int J Mol Sci 2022;23:14762.
12. Buettner R, Scholmerich J, Bollheimer LC. High-fat diets: modeling the metabolic disorders of human obesity in rodents. Obesity 2007;15:798–808.
13. Ito M, Suzuki J, Tsujioka S, et al. Longitudinal analysis of murine steatohepatitis model induced by chronic exposure to high-fat diet. Hepatol Res 2007;37:50–7.
14. Im YR, Hunter H, de Gracia Hahn D, et al. A systematic review of animal models of NAFLD finds high-fat, high-fructose diets most closely resemble human NAFLD. Hepatology 2021;74:1884–901.
15. Harris SE, Poolman TM, Arvaniti A, et al. The American lifestyle-induced obesity syndrome diet in male and female rodents recapitulates the clinical and transcriptomic features of nonalcoholic fatty liver disease and nonalcoholic steatohepatitis. Am J Physiol Gastrointest Liver Physiol 2020;319:G345–60.
16. Matsuzawa N, Takamura T, Kurita S, et al. Lipid-induced oxidative stress causes steatohepatitis in mice fed an atherogenic diet. Hepatology 2007;46:1392–403.

17. Charlton M, Krishnan A, Viker K, et al. Fast food diet mouse: novel small animal model of nash with ballooning, progressive fibrosis, and high physiological fidelity to the human condition. Am J Physiol Gastrointest Liver Physiol 2011;301: G825–34.

18. Sferruzzi-Perri AN, Lopez-Tello J, Napso T, et al. Exploring the causes and consequences of maternal metabolic maladaptations during pregnancy: lessons from animal models. Placenta 2020;98:43–51.

19. Pennington KA, van der Walt N, Pollock KE, et al. Effects of acute exposure to a high-fat, high-sucrose diet on gestational glucose tolerance and subsequent maternal health in mice. Biol Reprod 2017;96:435–45.

20. Musial B, Vaughan OR, Fernandez-Twinn DS, et al. A Western-style obesogenic diet alters maternal metabolic physiology with consequences for fetal nutrient acquisition in mice. J Physiol 2017;595:4875–92.

21. Lee SM, Jung YM, Choi ES, et al. Metabolic dysfunction-associated fatty liver disease and subsequent development of adverse pregnancy outcomes. Clin Gastroenterol Hepatol 2022;20:2542–50.

22. Lopez-Jaramillo P, Barajas J, Rueda-Quijano SM, et al. Obesity and preeclampsia: common pathophysiological mechanisms. Front Physiol 2018;9:1838.

23. Ajmera VH, Terrault NA, VanWagner LB, et al. Longer lactation duration is associated with decreased prevalence of non-alcoholic fatty liver disease in women. J Hepatol 2019;70:126–32.

24. Yeo E, Brubaker PL, Sloboda DM. The intestine and the microbiota in maternal glucose homeostasis during pregnancy. J Endocrinol 2022;253:R1–19.

25. Oben JA, Mouralidarane A, Samuelsson AM, et al. Maternal obesity during pregnancy and lactation programs the development of offspring non-alcoholic fatty liver disease in mice. J Hepatol 2010;52:913–20.

26. Ashino NG, Saito KN, Souza FD, et al. Maternal high-fat feeding through pregnancy and lactation predisposes mouse offspring to molecular insulin resistance and fatty liver. J Nutr Biochem 2012;23:341–8.

27. Marin V, Rosso N, Dal Ben M, et al. An animal model for the juvenile non-alcoholic fatty liver disease and non-alcoholic steatohepatitis. PLoS One 2016;11: e0158817.

28. de Paula Simino LA, de Fante T, Figueiredo Fontana M, et al. Lipid overload during gestation and lactation can independently alter lipid homeostasis in offspring and promote metabolic impairment after new challenge to high-fat diet. Nutr Metab 2017;14:16.

29. Saengnipanthkul S, Noh HL, Friedline RH, et al. Maternal exposure to high-fat diet during pregnancy and lactation predisposes normal weight offspring mice to develop hepatic inflammation and insulin resistance. Physiol Rep 2021;9:e14811.

30. Zhou Y, Peng H, Xu H, et al. Maternal diet intervention before pregnancy primes offspring lipid metabolism in liver. Lab Invest 2020;100:553–69.

31. Liang X, Yang Q, Fu X, et al. Maternal obesity epigenetically alters visceral fat progenitor cell properties in male offspring mice. J Physiol 2016;594:4453–66.

32. Wankhade UD, Zhong Y, Kang P, et al. Maternal high-fat diet programs offspring liver steatosis in a sexually dimorphic manner in association with changes in gut microbial ecology in mice. Sci Rep 2018;8:16502.

33. Chatzi L, Rifas-Shiman SL, Georgiou V, et al. Adherence to the Mediterranean diet during pregnancy and offspring adiposity and cardiometabolic traits in childhood. Pediatr Obes 2017;12(Suppl 1):47–56.

34. Ayonrinde OT, Adams LA, Mori TA, et al. Sex differences between parental pregnancy characteristics and nonalcoholic fatty liver disease in adolescents. Hepatology 2018;67:108–22.
35. Furse S, Koulman A, Ozanne SE, et al. Altered lipid metabolism in obese women with gestational diabetes and associations with offspring adiposity. J Clin Endocrinol Metab 2022;107:e2825–32.
36. Voerman E, Santos S, Patro Golab B, et al. Maternal body mass index, gestational weight gain, and the risk of overweight and obesity across childhood: an individual participant data meta-analysis. PLoS Med 2019;16:e1002744.
37. Manios Y, Birbilis M, Moschonis G, et al. Healthy Growth Study" group. childhood obesity risk evaluation based on perinatal factors and family sociodemographic characteristics: CORE index. Eur J Pediatr 2013;172:551–5.
38. Cinelli G, Fabrizi M, Ravà L, et al. Influence of maternal obesity and gestational weight gain on maternal and foetal lipid profile. Nutrients 2016;8:368.
39. Bianchi M, Alisi A, Fabrizi M, et al. Maternal intake of n-3 polyunsaturated fatty acids during pregnancy is associated with differential methylation profiles in cord blood white cells. Front Genet 2019;10:1050.
40. Bäckhed F, Roswall J, Peng Y, et al. Dynamics and stabilization of the human gut microbiome during the first year of life. Cell Host Microbe 2015;17:852.
41. Ferretti P, Pasolli E, Tett A, et al. Mother-to-infant microbial transmission from different body sites shapes the developing infant gut microbiome. Cell Host Microbe 2018;24:133–45.e5.
42. Nobili V, Bedogni G, Alisi A, et al. A protective effect of breastfeeding on the progression of non-alcoholic fatty liver disease. Arch Dis Child 2009;94:801–5.
43. Park Y, Sinn DH, Oh JH, et al. The association between breastfeeding and nonalcoholic fatty liver disease in parous women: a nation-wide cohort study. Hepatology 2021;74:2988–97.
44. Soderborg TK, Clark SE, Mulligan CE, et al. The gut microbiota in infants of obese mothers increases inflammation and susceptibility to NAFLD. Nat Commun 2018; 9:4462.
45. Soderborg TK, Carpenter CM, Janssen RC, et al. Gestational diabetes is uniquely associated with altered early seeding of the infant gut microbiota. Front Endocrinol 2020;11:603021.
46. Jian C, Carpén N, Helve O, et al. Early-life gut microbiota and its connection to metabolic health in children: perspective on ecological drivers and need for quantitative approach. EBioMedicine 2021;69:103475.
47. Mosca A, Panera N, Maggiore G, et al. From pregnant women to infants: non-alcoholic fatty liver disease is a poor inheritance. J Hepatol 2020;73:1590–2.
48. Ayonrinde OT, Oddy WH, Adams LA, et al. Infant nutrition and maternal obesity influence the risk of non-alcoholic fatty liver disease in adolescents. J Hepatol 2017;67:568–76.
49. Abeysekera KW, Orr JG, Madley-Dowd P, et al. Association of maternal prepregnancy BMI and breastfeeding with NAFLD in young adults: a parental negative control study. Lancet Reg Health Eur 2021;10:100206.
50. Panera N, Mandato C, Crudele A, et al. Genetics, epigenetics and transgenerational transmission of obesity in children. Front Endocrinol 2022;13:1006008.

The Interlink Between Metabolic-Associated Fatty Liver Disease and Polycystic Ovary Syndrome

Paulina Vidal-Cevallos, MD, Alejandra Mijangos-Trejo, MD,
Misael Uribe, MD, PhD, Norberto Chávez Tapia, MD, PhD*

KEYWORDS

- Polycystic ovary syndrome • Nonalcoholic fatty liver disease • Metabolic syndrome
- Insulin resistance • Lipid metabolism • Metabolic-associated fatty liver disease

KEY POINTS

- Polycystic ovary syndrome (PCOS) affects around 10% of women in the reproductive age group. Metabolic-associated fatty liver disease (MAFLD) is the leading cause of chronic liver disease worldwide and has a higher incidence in women with PCOS.
- MAFLD and PCOS share risk factors, including central obesity, insulin resistance, chronic low-grade inflammation, and hyperandrogenemia.
- Insulin resistance plays a pivotal role in the development of MAFLD and PCOS and interlinks these 2 entities.
- Lifestyle modifications, including diet, weight loss, and exercise, are the cornerstones of management for both entities.
- There is no approved pharmacological treatment of MAFLD; the need for effective therapies that can improve both PCOS and MAFLD is crucial.

INTRODUCTION

Polycystic ovary syndrome (PCOS) affects around 10% of women in the reproductive age group. PCOS is characterized by ovulatory dysfunction, hyperandrogenism, and/or polycystic ovarian morphology. PCOS is highly associated with metabolic syndrome and more commonly with obesity and insulin resistance. Metabolic-associated fatty liver disease (MAFLD) is the leading cause of chronic liver disease worldwide and has a higher incidence in women with PCOS.[1] Due to the common risk factors that these 2 diseases share, MAFLD and PCOS can coexist in women

Obesity and Digestive Disease Unit, Medica Sur Clinic and Foundation, Puente de Piedra 150, col. Toriello Guerra, Mexico City C.P. 14050, Mexico
* Corresponding author.
E-mail address: nchavezt@medicasur.org.mx

Endocrinol Metab Clin N Am 52 (2023) 533–545
https://doi.org/10.1016/j.ecl.2023.01.005
0889-8529/23/© 2023 Elsevier Inc. All rights reserved.

endo.theclinics.com

with high serum androgen levels, obesity, and insulin resistance.[2] The mechanisms involved in the development of MAFLD in women with PCOS are of high interest to clinicians for making evidence-based decisions. Management and therapeutic interventions are limited due to the presence of MAFLD in patients with PCOS.[3] Generally, clinicians recommend oral contraceptives and the antihyperglycemic drug metformin. Lifestyle interventions are also recommended in the clinical setting; however, the need for effective therapies that can improve both PCOS and MAFLD is crucial. Factors influencing successful outcomes are discussed in this review, along with the current clinical management of both conditions, challenges, and emerging therapies.

PATHOPHYSIOLOGY OF POLYCYSTIC OVARY SYNDROME

The pathogenesis of PCOS is multifactorial and includes genetic and environmental factors (**Table 1**).[3] Patients with PCOS have hypothalamic–pituitary-gonadal axis abnormalities, resulting in increased pulsatile release of gonadotropin-releasing hormone (GnRH). This leads to luteinizing hormone (LH) hypersecretion, which induces ovulary dysfunction and hyperandrogenism.[4] Although serum follicle-stimulating hormone (FSH) levels are generally normal, the follicles of patients with PCOS seem to be more resistant to FSH stimulation than those of healthy individuals.[4,5]

Although the growth of these follicles is arrested, the ovulatory dysfunction is characterized by increased follicular activation. Intraovarian factors involving follicular recruitment and growth, such as members of the transforming growth factor-beta family (ie, anti-Müllerian hormone [AMH], inhibins, activins, bone morphogenic proteins, and growth differentiation factors), and cytokines, also contribute to the abnormal follicle development and function seen in PCOS.[6]

High levels of AMH reduce the FSH sensitivity of individual ovarian follicles and block the conversion of androgens to estrogens via the inhibition of aromatase activity, thereby contributing to hyperandrogenism.[4,7] However, overstimulation of LH induces hypersecretion of androgens from theca cells, which show increased expression of several genes encoding steroidogenic enzymes.[4,8] Additionally, excess androgens

Table 1 Risk factors for polycystic ovary syndrome	
Genes	THADA FSHR INSR DENND1A
Endocrine-disrupting chemicals	Organochlorinated pesticides Industrial chemicals, plastics, and plasticizers fuels Bisphenol A Many other chemicals
Before birth	Mother affected with the syndrome Intrauterine exposure to excess androgens or glucocorticoids Intrauterine growth restriction
Childhood, peripuberty, and adolescence	Low socioeconomic status Insulin resistance Obesity, overweight, or rapid weight gain

Abbreviations: DENND1A, The domain differentially expressed in a normal and neoplastic domain containing 1A gene; FSHR, Follicle-stimulating hormone receptor gene; INSR, Insulin receptor gene; THADA, Thyroid adenoma-associated protein gene.

may reduce the sensitivity of the GnRH pulse generator to sex steroid inhibition in susceptible individuals.[7]

The described hormonal alterations result in menstrual abnormalities, anovulatory subfertility, and the accumulation of small antral follicles within the periphery of the ovary, giving it the characteristic polycystic morphology.[8]

Furthermore, animal studies and human data show that daughters born to mothers with PCOS have a 5-fold greater risk of the syndrome.[9] A strong association has been documented between genetic factors and PCOS; this has been demonstrated in heritability studies that report a high correlation (tetrachoric correlation of 0.71) between monozygotic twins with PCOS.[10]

Researchers have considered the potential environmental risk during the prenatal and postnatal periods. Experimental studies suggest that intrauterine exposure to excess androgens or glucocorticoids during certain critical periods of fetal development may determine the phenotypic expression of PCOS during adulthood.[9,11] One hypothesis suggests that intrauterine growth restriction may lead to increased prenatal exposure to androgens and glucocorticoids.[11,12]

It is also possible that some endocrine-disrupting chemicals, such as organochlorinated pesticides and industrial chemicals, plastics, plasticizers, and fuels, interfere with the biosynthesis, metabolism, and/or action of hormones. It is plausible that in utero exposure of human female fetuses to these androgen-like substances could result in PCOS in adulthood.[11]

High carbohydrate intake has been identified as a factor exacerbating PCOS, although the diet is probably not a cause of PCOS.[12] There is no evidence for causal effects of birth weight, adult height, age at menarche, blood pressure, or lipid fractions on PCOS.[13]

THE INTERLINK BETWEEN POLYCYSTIC OVARY SYNDROME AND METABOLIC-ASSOCIATED FATTY LIVER DISEASE

MAFLD and PCOS share risk factors, including central obesity, insulin resistance, chronic low-grade inflammation, and hyperandrogenemia.[14,15] Some reports indicate that 30% to 60% of patients with PCOS have obesity.[5] The prevalence of this syndrome in women with a body mass index (BMI) less than 25 kg/m^2 is 4.3%, whereas it is 14% in patients with a BMI less than 30 kg/m^2. Obesity is known to independently increase both insulin resistance and hyperandrogenism, thus exacerbating PCOS.[16]

Insulin resistance plays a pivotal role in the development of MAFLD and PCOS and interlinks these 2 entities.[1] Roughly 50% to 70% of women with PCOS have insulin resistance, which leads to compensatory hyperinsulinemia.[8,17] Excess insulin stimulates androgen production by ovarian theca cells and suppresses the hepatic production of sex hormone-binding globulin, which further contributes to androgen excess.[5,14]

Insulin resistance in adipose tissue results in accelerated lipolysis, causing an increased flow of free fatty acids to the liver, thus favoring hepatic fat accumulation.[18] Furthermore, hyperinsulinemia caused by insulin resistance leads to decreased mitochondrial fatty acid oxidation, generation of inflammation, necrosis, and fibrosis that ultimately leads to the progression of MAFLD.[1]

The distribution of adipose tissue is also important. It is known that visceral adipose tissue is more resistant to insulin than subcutaneous adipose tissue, and it also seems to be important in the pathogenesis of fatty liver disease due to increased portal flow of free fatty acids to the liver. Central adiposity is frequently present in individuals with PCOS, occurring independently of obesity.[18] Adipocytes and adipocyte function are aberrant in PCOS, favoring insulin resistance and subclinical inflammation.[4]

Other biological mechanisms support the association between the hyperandrogenemia of PCOS and the risk of MAFLD. Androgens can suppress low-density lipoprotein receptor gene transcription, thereby prolonging the half-life of very low-density lipoproteins (VLDLs) and LDL. As a result, lipids accumulate in the liver, and hyperandrogenic women become more prone to fatty liver.[19] Hyperandrogenemia can also increase androgen receptor transcripts and tumor necrosis factor-α release from mononuclear cells, inducing an inflammatory state that contributes to the development of MAFLD.[14,19]

THE COEXISTENCE OF POLYCYSTIC OVARY SYNDROME AND METABOLIC-ASSOCIATED FATTY LIVER DISEASE

The prevalence of PCOS using the Rotterdam criteria has been estimated to be 18% to 20%.[1,4] In contrast, MAFLD is one of the leading causes of chronic liver disease, with a prevalence of 6.3% to 33% with a median of 20% in the general population.[20] MAFLD and nonalcoholic steatohepatitis (NASH) are the most common hepatic diseases in women with PCOS.[14] In 2005, NAFLD was first associated with PCOS in a case report.[21] It has been found that women with PCOS have an increased risk of developing MAFLD compared with controls (odds ratio [OR] 2.49–3.31).[19,22]

In patients with MAFLD, the most common laboratory alteration, and often the only one, is elevated serum aminotransferase levels. Elevations of serum alkaline phosphatase and gamma-glutamyl transferase occur less frequently.[18] However, patients with MAFLD and NASH generally have normal liver enzymes, which lack the sensitivity to act as screening tests.[20]

DIAGNOSTIC WORKUP

PCOS should be suspected mainly in women with irregular menses, acne, alopecia, and hirsutism.[3] The diagnosis of PCOS is based on the variable presence of 3 specific elements: oligo-anovulation, androgen excess, and ultrasound evidence of polycystic ovarian morphology.[3,23] The Rotterdam criteria require that 2 of these 3 diagnostic criteria be met for diagnosis in adult women.[24]

Hyperandrogenism can be determined clinically by the presence of hirsutism and by biochemically measuring circulating androgen levels, including free and total testosterone levels and dehydroepiandrosterone sulfate. Ovulatory dysfunction is usually suspected based on a history of polymenorrhea or oligomenorrhea. To confirm ovulatory dysfunction, progesterone levels are measured on days 22 to 24 of the menstrual cycle, and AMH may be requested to assess increased antral follicle count. Finally, ovarian ultrasonography identifies polycystic morphology.[4,5]

Thyroid disease, hyperprolactinemia, and nonclassic form of congenital adrenal hyperplasia must always be excluded. In those patients with amenorrhea and atypical characteristics, it is recommended to rule out hypogonadotropic hypogonadism and Cushing disease, and to consider the evaluation of androgen-producing tumors.[3]

When the diagnosis of PCOS is confirmed, an oral glucose tolerance test and the measurement of serum glucose levels to assess insulin resistance should be performed.[5] Women with PCOS should also be routinely screened for abnormal liver enzyme levels and the presence of MAFLD because of the higher prevalence of fatty liver disease in this population, especially in patients with BMI greater than 25.[14,17]

Screening for MAFLD is necessary because most patients with MAFLD are asymptomatic at the time of diagnosis. Hepatomegaly may be the only physical finding. Therefore, the diagnosis is based on the evaluation of laboratory tests of liver function and/or imaging studies of the liver.[18]

A liver biopsy is the gold standard for diagnosing and staging of MAFLD. However, because biopsy is an invasive method associated with morbidity and is prone to sampling errors, several noninvasive methods have been proposed. Ultrasound is the most widely used first-line diagnostic modality, although it should be noted that ultrasound has limited sensitivity (80% in the presence of more than 30% of fatty infiltration) and its performance is suboptimal in individuals with BMI greater than 40 kg/m². [1,18,25] Another drawback of ultrasound is that its diagnostic performance is low in patients with mild steatosis (sensitivity of 61%–65%). [26]

Transient elastography measures liver stiffness noninvasively and has been used to identify fibrosis. Another less-used imaging tool is magnetic resonance elastography, which is also useful for measuring hepatic steatosis and fibrosis. [20] Elastography detects patients with steatosis and fibrosis with an area under receiver operating characteristic curve of 0.70 and 0.89, respectively. [27]

Diagnosis of MAFLD is based on histologic, imaging, and serological evidence of hepatic steatosis, plus one of the following 3 criteria: overweight/obesity, presence of type 2 diabetes mellitus, or evidence of the presence of at least 2 metabolic risk abnormalities (**Fig. 1**) but biopsy should be performed in very selected cases (ie, unclear diagnosis, research). [25]

COMPLICATION PROFILE, INCLUDING CARDIOVASCULAR RISKS

Classic cardiovascular risk factors, such as central adiposity, impaired glucose tolerance or diabetes mellitus, dyslipidemia, and hypertension, are frequently present in patients with PCOS and/or MAFLD. [18] MAFLD has been shown to increase cardiovascular risk (relative risk 3.13). [28]

Dyslipidemia occurs in 70% of women with PCOS. The most common atherogenic dyslipidemic manifestations in PCOS are hypertriglyceridemia, elevated levels of low-density lipoprotein cholesterol, very-low-density lipoprotein cholesterol, and low high-density lipoprotein cholesterol levels. [8,29]

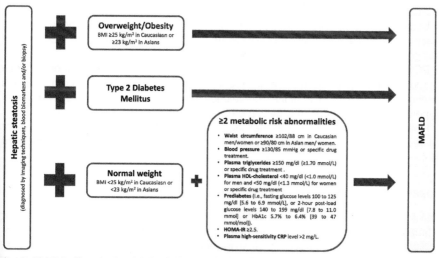

Fig. 1. MAFLD diagnostic criteria. (*Adapted from* Eslam M, Newsome PN, Sarin SK, et al. A new definition for metabolic dysfunction-associated fatty liver disease: An international expert consensus statement. *J Hepatol*. 2020;73(1):202-209.)

Many women with PCOS have hyperinsulinemia and insulin resistance. It has been found that insulin-mediated glucose disposal is lower in patients with PCOS than in matched controls.[4] Approximately 35% of women with PCOS have impaired glucose tolerance, and 7.5% to 10% have type 2 diabetes mellitus. There is a substantial increase in the incidence of diabetes associated with obesity among women with PCOS. However, PCOS increases the risk of diabetes even in lean women.[29]

Metabolic syndrome occurs in 33% to 47% of women with PCOS. Metabolic syndrome is an inflammatory atherothrombotic state with insulin resistance that elevates proinflammatory mediators, impairs endothelial function, reduces vasoreactivity, and promotes subclinical atherosclerosis. Consequently, women with PCOS have increased carotid intima–media thickness, coronary artery calcification, and subclinical vascular disease compared with women without PCOS.[4,8] A higher incidence of aortic calcification and arterial stenosis has been reported in patients with PCOS.[4] An increased prevalence of calcification of the coronary artery (46% vs 31%) and aorta (69% vs 55%) compared with controls has been observed.[30]

All women with PCOS should be checked for hypertension frequently because it often develops in patients with PCOS due to hyperaldosteronism consequent to activation of the renin–angiotensin system.[23,29] However, despite all the associations found, there is no evidence of whether these findings indicate a true increase in cardiovascular mortality.[18]

The risk of venous thromboembolism is also increased (OR 1.5) compared with BMI-matched controls, with the risk of venous thromboembolism being twice as high in women with PCOS taking oral contraceptives compared with the general population. In addition, women with PCOS taking combined oral contraceptives had an increased risk of venous thromboembolism compared with other contraceptives (OR 2.14).[31]

A meta-analysis found that women with PCOS have higher emotional distress than control populations (standardized mean difference [SMD] 0.60) for depression (SMD 0.49) and anxiety.[32] This syndrome has also even been associated with bipolar disorder, although the association may be with the disorder and specific treatments.[6,23]

Due to hyperestrogenic anovulation and hyperinsulinemia, women with PCOS have a 2-to-6-fold increased risk of endometrial cancer.[4,23] This increased risk applies to a subgroup of PCOS women with obesity because the risk is reduced but not eliminated when adjusted for BMI.[6] Moreover, patients with MAFLD have a higher incidence of malignant hepatic and extrahepatic tumors.[15]

PCOS causes anovulatory subfertility, and infertility is 15 times higher in these women. Furthermore, if they become pregnant, they have a higher risk of complications during pregnancy, and a higher prevalence of preeclampsia, pregnancy-induced hypertension, early pregnancy loss, preterm labor, and gestational diabetes.[4,33,34]

Finally, it must be considered that the presence of MAFLD causes hepatocellular injury and inflammation that produces fibrogenesis and culminates in the development of liver cirrhosis.[15]

CURRENT MANAGEMENT STRATEGIES AND THERAPEUTICS

The importance of early detection of MAFLD in patients with PCOS lies in the fact that a timely intervention in patients with steatosis or steatohepatitis can reduce the probability of disease progression.[18] Lifestyle modifications, including diet, weight loss, and exercise, alone or in combination with drug therapy, are the cornerstones of treatment. Weight loss of at least 3% to 5% of body weight has been shown to improve hepatic steatosis but a greater weight loss (up to 10%) may be needed to improve necroinflammation and fibrosis.[18,20] In a prospective study, it was found that the degree of weight loss was independently associated with histological improvement in fatty liver; 90% of the patients who lost more than 10% of their weight had resolution of steatohepatitis and 45% had regression of fibrosis. All patients with a weight loss greater than 10% had a decrease in steatosis.[35]

Similarly, lifestyle changes are also recommended for first-line treatment of PCOS, and 5% to 10% weight loss in 6 months is suggested (especially loss of abdominal fat).[3,23,34] It has been shown that weight reduction can improve insulin sensitivity, restore ovulation, reduce testosterone concentration, improve conception rates, and decrease spontaneous abortion rates.[34]

A Mediterranean diet has been recommended as improved liver fat has been seen even without weight loss. The Mediterranean diet is characterized by a reduced intake of carbohydrates (mainly sugars and refined carbohydrates) and monounsaturated fatty acids.[36] However, in polycystic ovarian syndrome, studies on the superiority of one type of diet over another are limited. The only thing that is recommended in these patients is caloric restriction.[23]

There is no approved pharmacological treatment of MAFLD,[1] although many agents have been tested, such as insulin sensitizers such as pioglitazone, hypolipidemic drugs and hepatoprotective agents, antioxidants, and anti-inflammatory agents (**Table 2**).[18] One meta-analysis found that pioglitazone decreases liver steatosis and improves ALT levels compared with controls.[37] Another meta-analysis showed that pioglitazone improved fibrosis compared with placebo (OR 1.66, $P = .01$, $I^2 = 0\%$).[38] Thiazolidinediones have been shown to reduce fasting insulin levels and improve insulin resistance in PCOS patients but are less effective in reducing BMI. However, due to their adverse effects they are not routinely recommended for the treatment of insulin resistance in PCOS.[4]

Metformin was found to be an ineffective treatment of liver steatosis because it was not superior to controls for any histological or biochemical outcome.[37] However, patients with PCOS taking metformin may experience small improvements in menstrual and ovulatory function.[5] Although metformin has only mild effects on cycle regularity and hyperandrogenism, it has potential use in insulin resistance and glucose improvement.[3] The use of metformin should be considered in women with metabolic disorders and for those who, despite lifestyle changes, do not achieve their goals.[23]

It has been observed that treatment with a glucagon like peptide-1 receptor agonist improves BMI and adiponectin levels in patients with MAFLD.[1] In addition, beneficial effects on liver enzymes and liver fat content have been demonstrated.[39] Liraglutide demonstrated a 39% reduction in hepatic fat content in patients with PCOS compared with placebo and a 5.6% reduction in body weight after 26 weeks of treatment.[40] Therefore, treatment with liraglutide is recommended for the treatment of obesity in patients with PCOS.[3]

Antioxidant agents target inflammation and oxidative stress. Vitamin E has been shown to reduce steatosis (54% vs 31%, $P = .001$) and inflammation (43% vs 19%, $P = .001$) compared with placebo but it does not influence liver fibrosis (see **Table 2**). Vitamin E is associated with a decrease in aminotransferase levels in subjects with fatty liver disease, and a daily dose of 800 IU is recommended. A special consideration is that vitamin E is not recommended to treat fatty liver disease in patients with diabetes.[1,20] Care should be taken with its administration because it has been associated with an increased risk of hemorrhagic stroke secondary to the antiplatelet effect at high doses.[39] In addition, the SELECT trial demonstrated an excess absolute risk of 1.6 for prostate cancer per 1000 person-years in older men receiving long-term vitamin E.[41]

Table 2 Pharmacological treatment of MAFLD		
Drug	Trial	Effects on MAFLD
Vitamin E	Sanyal et al,[42] 2010 PIVENS Study	Decreases steatohepatitis (43% vs 19%, $P = .001$), liver steatosis (54% vs 31%, $P = .001$), and improved alanine aminotransferase levels compared with placebo. No improvement in fibrosis scores
Pioglitazone	Sanyal et al,[42] 2010 PIVENS Study	Decreases steatohepatitis (34% vs 19%, $P = .04$), liver steatosis (69% vs 31%, $P = .001$), and improved ALT levels compared with placebo. No improvement in fibrosis scores
	Aithal et al,[43] 2008	Reduction of histological features of hepatocellular damage compared with placebo (32% vs 10%, $P = .005$)
	Belfort et al,[44] 2006	Decreases hepatic fat content (54% vs 0%, $P = .001$) and normalization of aspartate aminotransferase levels compared with placebo (58% vs 34%, $P = .001$)
Rosiglitazone	Ratziu et al,[45] 2008 FLIRT Trial	Improvement in steatosis (47% vs 16%; $P = .014$) and normalization of transaminase levels (38% vs 7%; $P = .005$) compared with placebo. No improvement in fibrosis
Metformin	Shields et al,[46] 2009	Did not show improvement in steatosis ($P = .23$) and fibrosis ($P = .44$)
	Haukeland (2009)	No demonstrated improvement in steatosis compared with placebo (38% vs 25%; $P = .52$)
Sitagliptin	Cui et al,[47] 2016	Not better in reducing liver fat measured by magnetic resonance at the end of the 24-wk treatment (18.1%–16.9%, $P = .27$) compared with placebo (16.6%–14.0%, $P = .07$)
Ursodeoxycholic acid	Leuschner et al,[48] 2010	Did not show improved histology in patients with steatohepatitis compared with placebo ($P = .061$)
Pentoxifylline	Zein et al,[49] 2011	Decreases steatosis (75% vs 19%; $P = .001$). No improvement in fibrosis

Finally, in patients with PCOS the use of combined contraceptives is recommended because they improve irregular menstrual cycles, hirsutism, and acne. When contraceptives are contraindicated or not well tolerated, antiandrogens could be considered to treat hirsutism and alopecia.[3,23]

However, the use of aromatase inhibitors such as letrozole is the treatment for ovulation induction in patients with PCOS who seek to become pregnant. In some cases, clomiphene may be used instead of letrozole.[3,34] In the case of patients resistant to fertility treatment, laparoscopic ovarian surgery could be a second-line therapy.[23] In vitro fertilization is the last option for treating infertility.[34]

We propose a management algorithm for patients with PCOS and MAFLD (**Fig. 2**).

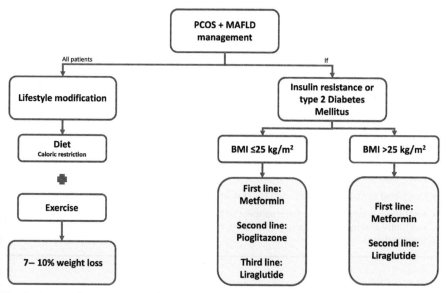

Fig. 2. Proposed management algorithm for patients with PCOS and MAFLD.

SUMMARY

There is a strong association between PCOS and MAFLD. It is recommended that patients with PCOS routinely undergo liver evaluation, including the measurement of aminotransferase levels and imaging tests to diagnose MAFLD. Early detection of MAFLD in patients with PCOS allows timely intervention, thereby reducing the risk of disease progression and cardiovascular complications.

The recommended initial treatment of MAFLD and PCOS is lifestyle modification, including diet, weight loss, and exercise. There is no approved pharmacological treatment of MAFLD. Among the treatments studied, we find mainly pioglitazone and vitamin E, which have been shown to reduce the degree of hepatic steatosis. However, no currently available treatment has been shown to improve fibrosis.

More research is needed to better understand the relationship between the 2 diseases and find therapeutic options to reduce cardiovascular risk and revert fibrosis.

CLINICS CARE POINTS

- MAFLD and PCOS can coexist in women with high serum androgen levels, obesity, and insulin resistance. Women with PCOS have an increased risk of developing MAFLD (OR 2.49–3.31).

- PCOS should be suspected mainly in women with irregular menses, acne, alopecia, and hirsutism. The diagnosis of PCOS is based on the presence of 2 of the following elements: oligoanovulation, androgen excess, and polycystic ovarian morphology.

- If PCOS is clinically suspected, laboratory tests should be ordered to confirm diagnosis: free and total testosterone levels, dehydroepiandrosterone sulfate, progesterone levels measured on days 22 to 24 of the menstrual cycle, and ovarian ultrasonography.

- Women with PCOS should also be routinely screened for MAFLD, especially in patients with BMI greater than 25.

- Diagnosis of MAFLD is based on histologic, imaging, and serological evidence of hepatic steatosis, plus one of the following 3 criteria: overweight/obesity, presence of type 2 diabetes mellitus, or evidence of the presence of at least 2 metabolic risk abnormalities.
- Due to hyperestrogenic anovulation and hyperinsulinemia, women with PCOS have a 2-to-6-fold increased risk of endometrial cancer.
- Lifestyle modifications, including calorie-restricted diet, weight loss, and exercise, alone or in combination with drug therapy, are the cornerstones of treatment. Weight loss of up to 10% improves necroinflammation and fibrosis.
- There is no approved pharmacological treatment of MAFLD. One meta-analysis found that pioglitazone decreases liver steatosis and improves ALT levels compared with controls. Another meta-analysis showed that pioglitazone improved fibrosis compared with placebo (OR 1.66).
- Combined contraceptives are used to treat irregular menstrual cycles, hirsutism, and acne.
- Metformin is ineffective for the treatment of liver steatosis and has only mild effects on cycle regularity and hyperandrogenism; however, it should be used to treat insulin resistance in these patients.

DECLARATION OF INTERESTS

This research received funding by Medica Sur Clinic and Foundation.

REFERENCES

1. Spremović Radenović S, Pupovac M, Andjić M, et al. Prevalence, risk factors, and pathophysiology of nonalcoholic fatty liver disease (NAFLD) in women with polycystic ovary syndrome (PCOS). Biomedicines 2022;10(1):131.
2. Rocha ALL, Faria LC, Guimarães TCM, et al. Non-alcoholic fatty liver disease in women with polycystic ovary syndrome: systematic review and meta-analysis. J Endocrinol Invest 2017;40(12):1279–88.
3. Hoeger KM, Dokras A, Piltonen T. Update on PCOS: consequences, challenges, and guiding treatment. J Clin Endocrinol Metab 2021;106(3):e1071–83.
4. Azziz R, Carmina E, Chen Z, et al. Polycystic ovary syndrome. Nat Rev Dis Primer 2016;2(1):16057.
5. Azziz R. Polycystic ovary syndrome. Obstet Gynecol 2018;132(2):321–36.
6. Dumesic DA, Oberfield SE, Stener-Victorin E, et al. Scientific Statement on the diagnostic criteria, epidemiology, pathophysiology, and molecular genetics of polycystic ovary syndrome. Endocr Rev 2015;36(5):487–525.
7. Catteau-Jonard S, Dewailly D. Pathophysiology of polycystic ovary syndrome: the role of hyperandrogenism. Front Horm Res 2013;40:22–7.
8. Goodarzi MO, Dumesic DA, Chazenbalk G, et al. Polycystic ovary syndrome: etiology, pathogenesis and diagnosis. Nat Rev Endocrinol 2011;7(4):219–31.
9. Risal S, Pei Y, Lu H, et al. Prenatal androgen exposure and transgenerational susceptibility to polycystic ovary syndrome. Nat Med 2019;25(12):1894–904.
10. Vink JM, Sadrzadeh S, Lambalk CB, et al. Heritability of polycystic ovary syndrome in a dutch twin-family study. J Clin Endocrinol Metab 2006;91(6):2100–4.
11. Diamanti-Kandarakis E, Bourguignon JP, Giudice LC, et al. Endocrine-disrupting chemicals: an endocrine society scientific statement. Endocr Rev 2009;30(4):293–342.

12. Merkin SS, Phy JL, Sites CK, et al. Environmental determinants of polycystic ovary syndrome. Fertil Steril 2016;106(1):16–24.

13. Zhu T, Goodarzi MO. Causes and consequences of polycystic ovary syndrome: insights from mendelian randomization. J Clin Endocrinol Metab 2022;107(3): e899–911.

14. Chen MJ, Ho HN. Hepatic manifestations of women with polycystic ovary syndrome. Best Pract Res Clin Obstet Gynaecol 2016;37:119–28.

15. Salva-Pastor N, Chávez-Tapia NC, Uribe M, et al. Understanding the association of polycystic ovary syndrome and non-alcoholic fatty liver disease. J Steroid Biochem Mol Biol 2019;194:105445.

16. Teede HJ, Joham AE, Paul E, et al. Longitudinal weight gain in women identified with polycystic ovary syndrome: results of an observational study in young women: weight gain and BMI in PCOS. Obesity 2013;21(8):1526–32.

17. Salva-Pastor N, López-Sánchez GN, Chávez-Tapia NC, et al. Polycystic ovary syndrome with feasible equivalence to overweight as a risk factor for non-alcoholic fatty liver disease development and severity in Mexican population. Ann Hepatol 2020;19(3):251–7.

18. Vassilatou E. Nonalcoholic fatty liver disease and polycystic ovary syndrome. World J Gastroenterol 2014;20(26):8351–63.

19. Wu J, Yao XY, Shi RX, et al. A potential link between polycystic ovary syndrome and non-alcoholic fatty liver disease: an update meta-analysis. Reprod Health 2018;15(1):77.

20. Naga C, Zobair Y, Joel EL. The diagnosis and management of non-alcoholic fatty liver disease: practice guideline by the american association for the study of liver diseases, american college of gastroenterology, and the american gastroentero-logical association. Hepatology 2012;55(6):2005–23.

21. Brown AJ, Tendler DA, McMurray RG. Polycystic ovary syndrome and severe nonalcoholic steatohepatitis: beneficial effect of modest weight loss and exercise on liver biopsy findings. Endocr Pract 2005;11(5):319–24.

22. Shengir M, Chen T, Guadagno E, et al. Non-alcoholic fatty liver disease in pre-menopausal women with polycystic ovary syndrome: A systematic review and meta-analysis. JGH Open 2021;5(4):434–45.

23. Teede HJ, Misso ML, Costello MF, et al. Recommendations from the international evidence-based guideline for the assessment and management of polycystic ovary syndrome. Hum Reprod 2018;33(9):1602–18.

24. Rotterdam ESHRE/ASRM-Sponsored PCOS Consensus Workshop Group. Revised 2003 consensus on diagnostic criteria and long-term health risks related to polycystic ovary syndrome. Fertil Steril 2004;81(1):19–25.

25. Eslam M, Newsome PN, Sarin SK, et al. A new definition for metabolic dysfunction-associated fatty liver disease: an international expert consensus statement. J Hepatol 2020;73(1):202–9.

26. Ferraioli G, Monteiro LBS. Ultrasound-based techniques for the diagnosis of liver steatosis. World J Gastroenterol 2019;25(40):6053–62.

27. Eddowes PJ, Sasso M, Allison M, et al. Accuracy of fibroscan controlled attenu-ation parameter and liver stiffness measurement in assessing steatosis and fibrosis in patients with nonalcoholic fatty liver disease. Gastroenterology 2019; 156(6):1717–30.

28. Musso G, Gambino R, Cassader M, et al. A meta-analysis of randomized trials for the treatment of nonalcoholic fatty liver disease. Hepatology 2010;52(1):79–104.

29. Osibogun O, Ogunmoroti O, Michos ED. Polycystic ovary syndrome and cardio-metabolic risk: opportunities for cardiovascular disease prevention. Trends Cardiovasc Med 2020;30(7):399–404.

30. Talbott EO, Zborowski JV, Rager JR, et al. Evidence for an association between metabolic cardiovascular syndrome and coronary and aortic calcification among women with polycystic ovary syndrome. J Clin Endocrinol Metab 2004;89(11): 5454–61.

31. Bird ST, Hartzema AG, Brophy JM, et al. Risk of venous thromboembolism in women with polycystic ovary syndrome: a population-based matched cohort analysis. Can Med Assoc J 2013;185(2):E115–20.

32. Veltman-Verhulst SM, Boivin J, Eijkemans MJC, et al. Emotional distress is a common risk in women with polycystic ovary syndrome: a systematic review and meta-analysis of 28 studies. Hum Reprod Update 2012;18(6):638–51.

33. Joham AE, Teede HJ, Ranasinha S, et al. Prevalence of infertility and use of fertility treatment in women with polycystic ovary syndrome: data from a large community-based cohort study. J Womens Health 2015;24(4):299–307.

34. Norman RJ, Dewailly D, Legro RS, et al. Polycystic ovary syndrome. Lancet 2007; 370(9588):685–97.

35. Vilar-Gomez E, Martinez-Perez Y, Calzadilla-Bertot L, et al. Weight loss through lifestyle modification significantly reduces features of nonalcoholic steatohepatitis. Gastroenterology 2015;149(2):367–78.e5.

36. Romero-Gómez M, Zelber-Sagi S, Trenell M. Treatment of NAFLD with diet, physical activity and exercise. J Hepatol 2017;67(4):829–46.

37. Rakoski MO, Singal AG, Rogers MAM, et al. Meta-analysis: insulin sensitizers for the treatment of non-alcoholic steatohepatitis: Meta-analysis: insulin sensitizers for NASH. Aliment Pharmacol Ther 2010;32(10):1211–21.

38. Musso G, Cassader M, Paschetta E, et al. Thiazolidinediones and advanced liver fibrosis in nonalcoholic steatohepatitis: a meta-analysis. JAMA Intern Med 2017; 177(5):633.

39. Rotman Y, Sanyal AJ. Current and upcoming pharmacotherapy for non-alcoholic fatty liver disease. Gut 2017;66(1):180–90.

40. Frøssing S, Nylander M, Chabanova E, et al. Effect of liraglutide on ectopic fat in polycystic ovary syndrome: a randomized clinical trial. Diabetes Obes Metab 2018;20(1):215–8.

41. Klein EA, Thompson IM, Tangen CM, et al. Vitamin E and the risk of prostate cancer: the selenium and Vitamin E cancer prevention trial (SELECT). JAMA 2011; 306(14):1549.

42. Sanyal AJ, Chalasani N, Kowdley KV, et al. Pioglitazone, Vitamin E, or Placebo for Nonalcoholic Steatohepatitis. N Engl J Med 2010;362(18):1675–85.

43. Aithal GP, Thomas JA, Kaye PV, et al. Randomized, placebo-controlled trial of pioglitazone in nondiabetic subjects with nonalcoholic steatohepatitis. Gastroenterology 2008;135(4):1176–84.

44. Belfort R, Harrison SA, Brown K, et al. A placebo-controlled trial of pioglitazone in subjects with nonalcoholic steatohepatitis. N Engl J Med 2006;355(22):2297–307.

45. Ratziu V, Giral P, Jacqueminet S, et al. Rosiglitazone for Nonalcoholic Steatohepatitis: one-year results of the randomized placebo-controlled fatty liver improvement with rosiglitazone therapy (FLIRT) trial. Gastroenterology 2008;135(1): 100–10.

46. Shields WW, Thompson KE, Grice GA, et al. The effect of metformin and standard therapy versus standard therapy alone in nondiabetic patients with insulin

resistance and nonalcoholic steatohepatitis (NASH): a pilot trial. Ther Adv Gastro-enterol 2009;2(3):157–63.
47. Cui J, Philo L, Nguyen P, et al. Sitagliptin vs. placebo for non-alcoholic fatty liver disease: a randomized controlled trial. J Hepatol 2016;65(2):369–76.
48. Leuschner UFH, Lindenthal B, Herrmann G, et al. High-dose ursodeoxycholic acid therapy for nonalcoholic steatohepatitis: a double-blind, randomized, placebo-controlled trial. Hepatology 2010;52(2):472–9.
49. Zein CO, Yerian LM, Gogate P, et al. Pentoxifylline improves nonalcoholic steato-hepatitis: a randomized placebo-controlled trial. Hepatology 2011;54(5):1610–9.

Management of Metabolic-Associated Fatty Liver Disease

Kirthika Venkatesan, MD, MPH[a,b], Nisha Nigil Haroon, MD[c,d],*

KEYWORDS

- Metabolic-associated fatty liver disease • Nonalcoholic fatty liver disease
- Nonalcoholic steatohepatitis • Lifestyle modifications • Pharmacotherapy
- Bariatric procedures

KEY POINTS

- Metabolic-associated fatty liver disease (MAFLD) is a novel term replacing nonalcoholic fatty liver disease.
- The prevalence of MAFLD is rising due to increasing rates of obesity and diabetes.
- There are no currently approved medical or surgical treatments for MAFLD.
- The leading cause of death in patients with MAFLD remains cardiometabolic complications.

INTRODUCTION

Metabolic-associated fatty liver disease (MAFLD), previously known as nonalcoholic fatty liver disease (NAFLD), is the most common cause of chronic liver disease in Western countries.[1] The prevalence of MAFLD is over 30%, which is increasing rapidly due to the rising incidence of obesity globally.[1,2] It is known that simple steatosis is often benign; however, progression to nonalcoholic steatohepatitis (NASH) increases the risk of mortality compared with the general population.[3]

Funding: This research did not receive any specific grant from funding agencies in the public, commercial, or not-for-profit sectors.
Competing Interests: None declared.
Author Contribution: K. Venkatesan: investigation, writing-original draft preparation, review and editing; N.N. Haroon: supervision, conceptualization, project administration, writing-original draft preparation, review and editing.
[a] Caribbean Medical University School of Medicine, 25 Pater Euwensweg, Willemstad, Curaçao; [b] Walden University, 650 South Exerter Street, Baltimore, MD 21202, USA; [c] Clinical Sciences Division, Northern Ontario School of Medicine, Sudbury, Ontario, Canada; [d] Health Sciences North Research Institute, Sudbury, Ontario, Canada
* Corresponding author. 115 Humber College Boulevard, Suite 610, Etobicoke, Ontario, Canada, M9V 1R8.
E-mail address: nnigilharoon@hsnsudbury.ca

Endocrinol Metab Clin N Am 52 (2023) 547–557
https://doi.org/10.1016/j.ecl.2023.02.002
0889-8529/23/© 2023 Elsevier Inc. All rights reserved.

endo.theclinics.com

The term MAFLD, developed in 2020, signifies a multisystem disorder compared with NAFLD which signifies liver disease only in the absence of alcohol use. Scientists concluded that MAFLD is a more appropriate term which addresses the metabolic aspect of fatty liver disease in the absence of excessive alcohol consumption.[1] This term identifies an additional cohort with hepatic steatosis and metabolic dysfunction who are not identified with the term NAFLD.[4]

The current management regimen for MAFLD is lifestyle modifications, management of associated underlying metabolic risk factors, and possibly pharmacologic interventions. Genetic and environmental factors modify the risk and progression of MAFLD.[5] Advanced MAFLD can lead to liver fibrosis and cirrhosis.[6] Currently, there are no Food and Drug Administration (FDA)-approved drugs for the treatment of MAFLD due to several limitations including difficulties in obtaining liver biopsies for histologic assessments, the extensive process of drug development, and inherent limitations of preclinical models. Therapeutic interventions aim to prevent further complications. Owing to the difficulty of implementing and maintaining lifestyle and diet modifications, new therapies are required. This review focuses on the currently recognized clinical management of MAFLD and targeted treatments using the evidence-based approaches.

SCREENING AND DIAGNOSIS
Diagnosis

Patients are required to have ≥5% of steatosis in hepatocytes and metabolic risk factors for a diagnosis of MAFLD. Excessive alcohol consumption (≥30 g per day for men and ≥20 g per day for women) or other chronic liver diseases must be excluded.[7]

Classically, patients are overweight/obese and/or have type 2 diabetes along with various abnormalities in biomarkers that signify MAFLD. There is a strong correlation between obesity and MAFLD. Patients may also have a normal body weight provided they meet at least two of the following parameters: (1) waist circumference ≥120 cm in Caucasian men and ≥88 cm in women (or ≥90 cm in Asian men and ≥80 cm in Asian women); (2) blood pressure ≥130/85 mm Hg or on hypertension drug treatment; (3) plasma triglycerides ≥150 mg/dL/≥2.3 mmol/L or on drug treatment; (4) plasma HDL less than 40 mg/dL/less than 1.03 mmol/L for men and less than 50 mg/dL/less than 1.3 mmol/L for women or on drug treatment; (5) prediabetes; (6) homeostasis model assessment of insulin resistance score ≥2.5; or (7) plasma high-sensitivity C-reactive protein level greater than 2 mg/L.[7] The diagnostic criteria for MAFLD are illustrated in **Fig. 1**.

Clinical Presentation

MAFLD usually presents in the fourth or fifth decade of life, although it can also occur during childhood.[8] Women have a greater risk of progression than men to advanced stages; however, men are more likely to have MAFLD.[9,10] There is a higher prevalence of MAFLD in Caucasian and Hispanic patients than in African American patients.[9] Patients with MAFLD often have diabetes, hypertension, dyslipidemia, and obesity.[6]

Patients are often asymptomatic unless they reach advanced liver disease where they will present with jaundice, fatigue, and right upper quadrant abdominal pain. Patients may present with obesity and/or features of insulin resistance, such as acanthosis nigricans and skin tags. Laboratory work normally shows mildly elevated liver enzymes. Hepatomegaly is evident in 10% of cases.[11] There is an 11% risk of progression to hepatocellular carcinoma in patients with MAFLD. Known predictors for malignant transformation include advanced age, male sex, and Hispanic ethnicity.

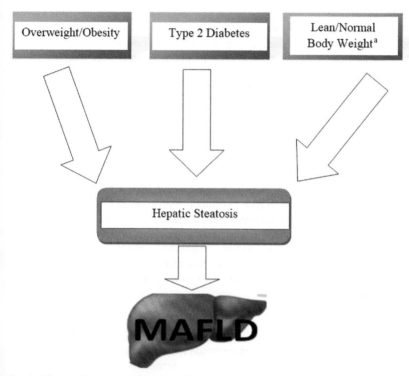

Fig. 1. Diagnostic criteria of MAFLD. [a]Must also meet at least two of the following parameters: 1. Waist circumference ≥120 cm in Caucasian men and ≥ 88 cm in women (or ≥ 90 cm in Asian men and ≥ 80 cm in Asian women. 2. Blood pressure ≥ 130/85 mmHg or on hypertension drug treatment. 3. Plasma triglycerides ≥ 150 mg/dL or its drug treatment. 4. Plasma HDL < 40 mg/dL for men and < 50 mg/dL for women or its drug treatment. 5. Prediabetes. 6. Homeostasis model assessment of insulin resistance score ≥ 2.5 7. Plasma high-sensitivity C-reactive protein level > 2 mg/L

Radiological Markers

The degree of liver fibrosis is considered a major factor in liver-related morbidity and mortality. The MAFLD fibrosis score, the aspartate transaminase (AST)-to-platelet ratio index, and the fibrosis-4 index are noninvasive clinic laboratory parameters to determine significant or advanced fibrosis in patients with fatty liver disease. These scores are reliable in providing negative predictive values used to exclude advanced fibrosis but can also yield false negative results. Their scores vary across a patient's lifespan and are different across ethnicities. Overall, it is only a modest diagnostic tool for gauging the degree of liver fibrosis.[12]

Biomarkers

Novel biomarkers for the diagnosis of MAFLD have emerged but are not widely used in clinical practice. For example, the enhanced liver fibrosis (ELF) panel is a noninvasive test to determine liver fibrosis. It includes serum biomarkers such as tissue inhibitor of matrix metalloproteinases-1, aminoterminal propeptide of procollagen type III, and hyaluronic acid. Based on the serum concentrations of these biomarkers, an ELF score is generated indicating the histologic stage of fibrosis which is a reliable marker across several studies. The ELF score is efficient and may reduce the need for a confirmatory liver biopsy.[13] Furthermore, macrophages are crucial biomarkers in the role of liver fibrosis. Soluble CD163, a macrophage activation marker, predicts advanced fibrosis. A macrophage-derived deaminase also can predict advanced fibrosis.[12]

Hepatokines are hormone-like proteins produced by hepatocytes and have been implicated in the onset and progression of MAFLD. These include fetuin-A, fetuin-B, angiopoietin-like proteins and fibroblast growth factor 21. These biomarkers are elevated in fatty liver disease and are promising as noninvasive biomarkers for MAFLD.[14,15] Although multiple genetic variants have been discovered relating to MAFLD, none are used as biomarkers due to its lack of consensus and health disparities. Another limitation of the use of genetic variants in MAFLD is the lack of its application at the individual level.

Liver Enzymes

Elevated liver enzymes are noted in 20% of patients with MAFLD. Alanine aminotransferase (ALT) and AST levels can be normal or mildly elevated around 1.5 to 2 times the upper standard limit with an AST/ALT ratio of less than 1. Hence, these enzymes are not reliable markers of fatty liver disease. In addition, alkaline phosphatase and gamma-glutamyl transpeptidase (GGT) levels may also vary. Body mass index (BMI) is also not a reliable indicator of the extent of elevation in liver enzymes.[16]

Imaging

Hepatic steatosis is detected using ultrasonography, computed tomography (CT) scan, magnetic resonance imaging (MRI), proton magnetic resonance spectroscopy, and liver biopsy. Ultrasound is the most common method to detect steatosis as it is noninvasive and efficient. However, ultrasound has limited sensitivity and specificity for detecting MAFLD in patients with obesity, especially with a liver fat content less than 12.5%.[17]

A fibroscan may also be used to measure liver stiffness (a marker for fibrosis). Transient elastography/fibroscan and acoustic radiation force impulse (ARFI) elastography can be combined with ultrasound to measure the extent of liver stiffness. The stiffness of a normal liver is between 6.5 and 7 kPa and anything higher suggests increased liver stiffness or steatosis. ARFI measures shearing velocity. The normal velocity of the liver is 1 m/s, which decreases once there is fatty infiltration.

Non-contrast CT scans demonstrate reduced attenuation in livers with steatosis. It is accurate in diagnosing steatosis of greater than 30% with 100% specificity and 82% sensitivity. As a general rule, the degree of decrease in attenuation on unenhanced CT is the best determinant of the degree of steatosis in the liver. MRI is a radiation-free alternative; however, it is costly and time-consuming. MRI offers more accurate detection of microscopic hepatic steatosis.

Liver biopsy is considered the gold standard for MAFLD diagnosis as noninvasive procedures cannot distinguish between simple hepatic steatosis and MAFLD.[16] The efficacy of liver biopsy has a risk of sampling errors, and there is poor consensus among pathologists along with the associated procedural risks.[12]

Grading and Staging of Metabolic-Associated Fatty Liver Disease

MAFLD is graded into three categories: Grade 1, Grade 2, and Grade 3. This is classified based on the degree of steatosis, ballooning, intralobular inflammation, and portal inflammation. Refer to **Table 1** for the grading of MAFLD.[18] The stages are based on the degree of steatosis, ballooning, and inflammation. There is also a staging system based on the location and extent of fibrosis. Stage 1 involves perisinusoidal fibrosis in zone 3, stage 2 involves portal fibrosis, and stage 3 extends to involve

Table 1
Grading of MAFLD

Grading	Steatosis	Ballooning	Intralobular Inflammation	Portal Inflammation
Grade 1 (mild)	Up to 66%	Occasional in Zone 3	Dispersed polymorphs with or without lymphocytes	Mild or none
Grade 2 (moderate)	Any degree	Predominantly in Zone 3	Polymorphs and chronic inflammation	Mild to moderate
Grade 3 (severe)	Panacinar	Ballooning and disarray in Zone 3	Dispersed polymorphs with or without chronic inflammation	Mild or moderate

bridging fibrosis. Stage 1 is subclassified into three categories: stage 1A (mild perisinusoidal fibrosis in zone 3); stage 1B (moderate perisinusoidal fibrosis in zone 3), and stage 1C (only portal/periportal fibrosis).[18]

The NAFLD activity score is used for characterizing the full spectrum of MAFLD and to calculate the histologic changes over time. However, its scores have also been used to diagnose MAFLD, especially scores greater than 5 are classified as diagnostic of MAFLD. It is calculated as the unweighted sum of the scores for steatosis (0–3), lobular inflammation (0–3), and ballooning (0–2).

CLINICAL MANAGEMENT OF MAFLD
Lifestyle Modifications

Patients with morbid obesity are more likely to have severe fibrosis and cirrhosis. Hence, weight loss is suggested. Owing to the lack of any approved medications for MAFLD treatment, lifestyle modifications (diet and exercise) are recommended.[19] Success with lifestyle modifications may be challenging due to the lack of compliance; hence, health care providers often prefer medications. Weight loss of 3% to 5% via lifestyle modifications has been shown to improve steatosis with the reversal of hepatic insulin resistance. Improvement in liver fibrosis has been found with weight loss of greater than 10% through lifestyle management. Nutritional modifications with a weight loss of greater than 5% have been shown to improve MAFLD. Dietary modifications include reducing carbohydrate intake, added sugars, and saturated fat. Intermittent fasting also has been shown to improve MAFLD. The ultimate goal is to aim for calorie deficit. Mediterranean diet is often preferred in patients with MAFLD due to its low glycemic effects and cardiovascular benefits.[20]

Exercise improves all-cause morbidity and mortality associated with MAFLD. Aerobic exercise and resistance training reduce intrahepatic triglyceride content. Aerobic exercise for 150 to 300 min/wk of moderate-intensity or 75 to 150 min/wk of high-intensity exercise with resistance training with a weight loss greater than 5% can improve hypertension, obstructive sleep apnea, diabetes, and dyslipidemia in patients with MAFLD.[20]

Underlying Comorbidities

MAFLD occurs due to multiple factors including adverse lifestyle habits and genetic factors. A sedentary lifestyle, poor dietary choices, and lack of preventative care all cause an increased risk of metabolic syndrome ultimately leading to MAFLD and an increased risk of hepatocellular carcinoma. Management of underlying comorbidities includes engaging in a healthy lifestyle. Weight loss and a diabetic diet are highly advised to prevent progression to advanced liver disease due to the decrease in fat accumulation and insulin resistance.

Pregnant Women and Children

MAFLD has adverse effects on maternal and fetal health. Its prevalence in pregnancy has nearly tripled over the past 10 years.[21] The risk factors contributing to the onset of MAFLD are limited; however, preexisting history of diabetes, obesity, and dyslipidemia contributes to an increased risk of MAFLD during pregnancy. Mothers with MAFLD have an increased risk of maternal hypertension, maternal obesity, higher risk of preterm delivery, and postpartum hemorrhage. Maternal obesity is also linked to a large gestational age fetus leading to an increased risk of delivery complications such as shoulder dystocia. Maternal MAFLD also increases the risk of gestational diabetes mellitus which is linked to altered infant metabolism posing an increased risk of diabetes and MAFLD later in the infant's life. In-utero exposure to disrupted maternal metabolism can increase the risk of childhood MAFLD through placental transfer. Specifically, the transfer of fatty acids and excess maternal glucose can lead to fetal ectopic lipids leading to a predisposition of pediatric obesity and insulin resistance. Hence, maternal metabolic complications should be managed before conception and during pregnancy.[21]

A safe diagnostic method for MAFLD detection in pregnant women is challenging. It is not suitable and is invasive to conduct a liver biopsy in a pregnant woman in the absence of symptoms. Although the specificity and sensitivity of ultrasound are limited in patients with obesity, it is the preferred method for MAFLD detection in pregnant women.[22] Further research is required to establish an accurate diagnostic tool for pregnant women with MAFLD. Lifestyle modifications during the postpartum period are crucial for reducing the complications associated with MAFLD in the next pregnancy.[20]

Around 2.6% to 9.6% of children and adolescents have MAFLD. The prevalence of pediatric MAFLD has increased from 19.34 million in 1990 to 29.49 million in 2017.[23] Prenatal risk factors include maternal obesity and gestational diabetes. Postnatal risk factors include obesity, hyperinsulinemia, insulin resistance, and a diet high in fructose, carbohydrates, and fat.

MAFLD has become the most common cause of chronic liver disease in children and adolescents. Patients with childhood-onset MAFLD are at an increased risk of progressive disease. In addition, children and adolescents commonly present with neuropsychiatric symptoms and overall poor quality of life. Those with a history of intellectual disability have a higher risk of developing MAFLD. Children less than 10 years of age with hepatic steatosis have an increased prevalence of secondary causes (ie, hepatitis C) and must be screened.[23]

The histologic differences of MAFLD between children and adults are: (1) adult hepatic steatosis affects zone 3 and children's steatosis affects zone 1 and 3; (2) the severity of steatosis is higher in children but mild to moderate in adults; (3) adult patients are prone to lobular inflammation, but children usually have portal inflammation; and (4) fibrosis in adult patients is described as pericellular with collagen strands around the damaged hepatocytes contributing to the "chicken wire" appearance, whereas in children, it is portal–periportal fibrosis.[23]

Management of MAFLD in children and adolescents includes education, lifestyle modifications, family support, and psychological support therapies. A diet low in free sugar with probiotics and aerobic and resistance training are recommended with ≥ 60 min/session at least three times a week. If weight loss is inadequate, referral to an intensive weight loss program or initiation of pharmacotherapy is advised (ie, statins, and drugs with weight loss potential). If all other measures fail, bariatric surgery may help in advanced steatohepatitis in adolescents with comorbidities and moderate/severe obesity.[23]

CLINICAL MANAGEMENT OF ADVANCED MAFLD
Pharmacotherapies

There are currently no FDA-approved treatments for MAFLD. If lifestyle modifications are not sustainable, anti-obesity medications are added (ie, orlistat, glucagon-like peptide-1 (GLP-1) analogues, and naltrexone/bupropion). The average hemoglobin A1C (HbA1c) reduction in patients taking GLP-1 receptor agonists is between 0.66% and 2.3%, and the mean weight loss achieved is between 2.0 and 11.4 kg. [24]

Tirzepatide is a novel antidiabetic drug with both GLP-1 and glucose-dependent insulinotropic polypeptide effects. It has cardiovascular benefits and is highly effective in reducing body weight, with improvements in lipid profiles in patients with type 2 diabetes. Weight loss can range from 15% to 20.9% from baseline with 5 to 15 mg of tirzepatide per week. The main side effects are mostly gastrointestinal-related such as nausea, vomiting, diarrhea, and constipation. Tirzepatide is promising in reducing MAFLD; however, further research is necessary to identify the extent of improvement.[25]

Sodium-glucose cotransporter type-2 inhibitors are recognized for their antihyperglycemic effects, eliminating uric acid from the body, and promoting weight loss. It promotes weight loss through improvements in insulin resistance, increased body temperature, and metabolism. It also reduces free fatty acid oxidation and lipogenesis in the liver.[26] The GLP-1 receptor analogues affect the gastrointestinal system to delay gastric emptying. As a result, patients have suppressed appetite resulting in weight loss. GLP-1 receptor analogues should be used with caution or avoided in patients with type 1 diabetes, diabetic retinopathy, history of pancreatitis, and personal or family history of medullary thyroid carcinoma or history of MEN syndrome. Other medications such as naltrexone and bupropion combinations (ie, Contrave) are also effective in weight loss but are avoided in patients with a history of opioid use, eating disorders, and seizures.

Metformin is often the first medication for patients with type 2 diabetes. It reduces insulin resistance and improves glycemic profile while achieving weight loss. It works on the liver to reduce gluconeogenesis. It improves MAFLD through improvement in liver enzymes and lipid profile. Side effects include diarrhea, vitamin B12 deficiency, and lactic acidosis. Metformin has been shown to reduce the effects of high-fat-induced hepatic steatosis in maternal rats, fetal liver cell apoptosis, and intestinal inflammation. Although metformin is safe during pregnancy, there are no human studies on its routine use in pregnant women with MAFLD.[27]

Owing to limited evidence of metformin use for MAFLD in patients without type 2 diabetes, it is not recommended as a therapeutic agent for this population. However, it is recommended for those with type 2 diabetes.[28]

Vitamin E use can lead to improved liver enzymes and histology of MAFLD with steatohepatitis in adults. However, a high dose of vitamin E is associated with worsening insulin resistance; hence, it is not advised in patients with type 2 diabetes and those with fibrosis.[19] Obeticholic acid (OCA) is a farnesoid X receptor agonist approved for the treatment of primary biliary cholangitis. Bile acids bind to the G-protein-coupled bile acid receptors and activate the farnesoid X receptor which regulates bile acid synthesis, glucose, and lipid metabolism. This reduces liver inflammation and fibrosis and improves insulin sensitivity.[29]

Statins may also be used in patients with MAFLD with cardiovascular complications. Statins are associated with a significant improvement in liver steatosis, inflammation, fibrosis, and reduce risk of hepatocellular carcinoma.[30,31] In summary, the American Association of Clinical Endocrinology (AACE) guidelines 2022 do not recommend the use of metformin, Dipeptidyl peptidase-4 (DPP-4) inhibitors, acarbose, and insulins due to a lack of evidence in improving hepatic inflammation and steatosis.[19]

Bariatric Surgery

If the combination of lifestyle modifications and medications is unsuccessful, bariatric surgery is considered in obese patients (with a BMI of 35–39.9 with one or more severe medical conditions or BMI $\geq$40).[32] As per the AACE guidelines, bariatric surgery is suggested for patients with MAFLD (especially with type 2 diabetes) with a BMI of 35 or more.[19]

Approximately 20% of patients with MAFLD will develop cirrhosis during their lifetimes.[33] Hence, bariatric surgery improves symptoms of metabolic syndrome and liver abnormailities in the majority of obese patients with MAFLD, such as grade of steatosis, hepatic inflammation, and fibrosis.[33] These changes are not only dominated by weight loss but also through changes in the gut microbiota. The two commonly practiced bariatric surgeries include Roux-en-Y gastric bypass and sleeve gastrectomy. In the latter, the fundus of the stomach is removed, and in the former, a new pouch is created and joined with the small intestine. Both types of procedures are effective in weight loss; however, Roux-en-Y gastric bypass involves changes in bile acid reabsorption.[34,35] Roux-en-Y gastric bypass is an effective bariatric surgical procedure for patients with MAFLD as it achieves greater weight loss than any other bariatric surgical procedure. However, sleeve gastrectomy is superior to Roux-en-Y gastric bypass in reducing ALT, AST, GGT, high-density lipoprotein (HDL), and triglyceride levels and demonstrates complete MAFLD resolution on ultrasound on those who have achieved greater than 50% weight loss.[26] Studies demonstrate such improvement in MAFLD within the first 8 to 10 weeks after bariatric surgery. This is a phase when no significant weight loss will be achieved. This could be due to the acute structural and endocrine changes involved in the reduction of metabolic syndrome.

In patients with cirrhosis, bariatric surgery can lead to malabsorption and significant morbidity and mortality, including acute-on-chronic liver failure. Other complications include anastomosis disruption and dumping syndrome. Portal hypertension is a contraindication for surgery. Sleeve gastrectomy is preferred in patients with cirrhosis as it reduces the risk of malabsorption. There is no clear indication of which bariatric surgical procedure is best for patients with severe, decompensated cirrhosis.[36] Before bariatric surgery, patients may need to lose a certain amount of weight, for which bariatric endoscopy may be used. Although the data on its prognosis are limited, it may help improve insulin resistance and lipid profiles.

Endo-barrier treatment involves placing a device in the duodenum that mimics the effects of gastric bypass, resulting in weight loss and improvement in glycemic profile. The linear device bypasses the duodenum to deliver food contents directly into the jejunum. Once implanted, it can stay there for a maximum of 12 months after which the device is explanted. The procedure can result in moderate weight loss and improvement in glycemic control. Common side effects include abdominal pain and nausea. Liver abscess is the most serious complication with most cases being reported toward the time of explantation.[37]

Current Clinical Trials

Several drugs are in phase 2 and 3 clinical trials for MAFLD treatment. Lanifibranor, a peroxisome proliferator–activated receptor (pan-PPAR) agonist, is currently in phase 2 trials and shows promising results as a new therapeutic option for patients with

MAFLD with fibrosis. OCA has demonstrated clinically significant improvements in the histology of patients with MAFLD. None of these medications are safe for pregnant women with MAFLD.[21]

Areas of Uncertainty/Emerging Concepts

Future studies should focus on medications that target adipose tissue biology to decrease triglyceride accumulation, insulin resistance, and lipotoxicity. Furthermore, research on pregnant women is limited and appropriate diagnostic and therapeutic options need to be developed in this population to improve maternal and fetal health. Clinical trials can offer new insight into emerging therapeutic measures for MAFLD.

SUMMARY

MAFLD is rising along with obesity and type 2 diabetes mellitus. The inflammatory state caused by pro-inflammatory cytokines in the liver contributes to fatty liver disease ultimately leading to liver cirrhosis. Genetic factors and environmental influences play roles in the onset and progression of MAFLD. Although there are no currently approved treatments for MAFLD, lifestyle modifications and reduction in insulin resistance can improve if not reverse MAFLD. Bariatric surgery has been shown to improve liver enzymes and overall MAFLD symptoms through weight loss and gut microbiome changes. Further research is required in terms of diagnostic accuracy in patients with obesity and pregnant women and the treatment efficacy of novel clinical trials.

CLINICS CARE POINTS

- Practitioners must educate patients with diabetes, obesity, and hypercholesterolemia regarding their risk of metabolic-associated fatty liver disease (MAFLD).

- There is no Food and Drug Administration-approved drug treatment for MAFLD; however, weight loss and an active lifestyle are encouraged to reduce the progression of MAFLD to cirrhosis.

- Pregnant women with a risk of MAFLD should not be advised to lose weight during pregnancy, rather they should be advised to choose healthier food options and stay active.

REFERENCES

1. Eslam M, Sanyal AJ, George J, International Consensus Panel. MAFLD: A Consensus-Driven Proposed Nomenclature for Metabolic-Associated Fatty Liver Disease. Gastroenterology 2020;158(7):1999–2014.e1.
2. Powell EE, Wong VW, Rinella M. Non-alcoholic fatty liver disease. Lancet 2021; 397(10290):2212–24.
3. European Association for the Study of the Liver (EASL), European Association for the Study of Diabetes (EASD), European Association for the Study of Obesity (EASO). EASL-EASD-EASO Clinical Practice Guidelines for the management of non-alcoholic fatty liver disease. J Hepatol 2016;64:1388–402.
4. Nguyen VH, Le MH, Cheung RC, et al. Differential clinical characteristics and mortality outcomes in persons with NAFLD and/or MAFLD. Clin Gastroenterol Hepatol 2021;19(10):2172–81.
5. Jonas W, Schürmann A. Genetic and epigenetic factors determining NAFLD risk. Mol Metab 2021;50:101111.

6. Hagström H, Talbäck M, Andreasson A, et al. Ability of noninvasive scoring systems to identify individuals in the population at risk for severe liver disease. Gastroenterology 2020;158:200–14.
7. Drożdż K, Nabrdalik K, Hajzler W, et al. Metabolic-Associated Fatty Liver Disease (MAFLD), Diabetes, and Cardiovascular Disease: Associations with Fructose Metabolism and Gut Microbiota. Nutrients 2021;14(1):103.
8. Hegarty R, Singh S, Bansal S, et al. NAFLD to MAFLD in adults but the saga continues in children: an opportunity to advocate change. J Hepatol Apr 2021;74(4): 991–2.
9. Balakrishnan M, Patel P, Dunn-Valadez S, et al. Women Have a Lower Risk of Nonalcoholic Fatty Liver Disease but a Higher Risk of Progression vs Men: A Systematic Review and Meta-analysis. Clin Gastroenterol Hepatol 2021;19(1): 61–71.e15.
10. Riazi K, Swain MG, Congly SE, et al. Race and Ethnicity in Non-Alcoholic Fatty Liver Disease (NAFLD): A Narrative Review. Nutrients; 2022;14(21):4556.
11. Stengel JZ, Harrison SA. Nonalcoholic Steatohepatitis: Clinical Presentation, Diagnosis, and Treatment. Gastroenterol Hepatol 2006;2(6):440–9.
12. Alharthi J, Eslam M. Biomarkers of Metabolic (Dysfunction)-associated Fatty Liver Disease: An Update. J Clin translational Hepatol 2022;10(1):134–9.
13. Kennedy OJ, Parkes J, Tanwar S, et al. The Enhanced Liver Fibrosis (ELF) Panel: Analyte Stability Under Common Sample Storage Conditions Used in Clinical Practice. The J Appl Lab Med 2017;1(6):720–8.
14. Kim TH, Hong DG, Yang YM. Hepatokines and non-alcoholic fatty liver disease: linking liver pathophysiology to metabolism. Biomedicines 2021;9(12):1903.
15. Martin AR, Kanai M, et al. Clinical use of current polygenic risk scores may exacerbate health disparities. Nat Genet 2019;51(4):584–91.
16. Milić S, Lulić D, Štimac D. Non-alcoholic fatty liver disease and obesity: biochemical, metabolic and clinical presentations. World J Gastroenterol 2014;20(28): 9330–7.
17. Bril F, Ortiz-Lopez C, Lomonaco R, et al. Clinical value of liver ultrasound for the diagnosis of nonalcoholic fatty liver disease in overweight and obese patients. Liver Int 2015;35(9):2139–46.
18. Takahashi Y, Fukusato T. Histopathology of nonalcoholic fatty liver disease/nonalcoholic steatohepatitis. World J Gastroenterol 2014;20(42):15539–48.
19. Cusi K, Isaacs S, Barb D, et al. American Association of Clinical Endocrinology Clinical Practice Guideline for the Diagnosis and Management of Nonalcoholic Fatty Liver Disease in Primary Care and Endocrinology Clinical Settings: Co-Sponsored by the American Association for the Study of Liver Diseases (AASLD). Endocr Pract 2022;28(5):528–62.
20. Jeeyavudeen MS, Khan SKA, Fouda S, et al. Management of metabolic-associated fatty liver disease: The diabetology perspective. World J Gastroenterol 2023;29(1):126–43.
21. Fouda S, Vennikandam MM, Pappachan JM, et al. Pregnancy and Metabolic-associated Fatty Liver Disease: A Clinical Update. J Clin translational Hepatol 2022;10(5):947–54.
22. Dyah AA, Rahadina R. Metabolic-associated fatty liver disease and adverse maternal and fetal outcomes: a systematic review and meta-analysis. Clin Exp Hepatol 2021;7(3):305–11.
23. Ramírez-Mejía MM, Díaz-Orozco LE, Barranco-Fragoso B, et al. A Review of the Increasing Prevalence of Metabolic-Associated Fatty Liver Disease (MAFLD) in

Children and Adolescents Worldwide and in Mexico and the Implications for Public Health. Med Sci monitor 2021;27:e934134.

24. Fonseca VA, Alvarado-Ruiz R, Raccah D, et al. Efficacy and safety of the once-daily GLP-1 receptor agonist lixisenatide in monotherapy: a randomized, double-blind, placebo-controlled trial in patients with type 2 diabetes (GetGoal-Mono). Diabetes care 2012;35(6):1225–31.

25. Nauck MA, D'Alessio DA. Tirzepatide, a dual GIP/GLP-1 receptor co-agonist for the treatment of type 2 diabetes with unmatched effectiveness regrading glycaemic control and body weight reduction. Cardiovasc diabetology 2022;21(1):169.

26. Androutsakos T, Nasiri-Ansari N, Bakasis AD, et al. SGLT-2 Inhibitors in NAFLD: Expanding Their Role beyond Diabetes and Cardioprotection. Int J Mol Sci 2022;23(6):3107.

27. Huang SW, Ou YC, Tang KS, et al. Metformin ameliorates maternal high-fat diet-induced maternal dysbiosis and fetal liver apoptosis. Lipids Health Dis 2021; 20(1):100.

28. Lian J, Fu J. Efficacy of Various Hypoglycemic Agents in the Treatment of Patients With Nonalcoholic Liver Disease With or Without Diabetes : A Network Meta-Analysis. Front Endocrinol 2021;12:649018.

29. Thomas C, Pellicciari R, Pruzanski, et al. Targeting bile-acid signalling for metabolic diseases. Nat Rev Drug Discov 2008;7(8):678–93.

30. Pose E, Trebicka J, Mookerjee RP, et al. Statins: Old drugs as new therapy for liver diseases? J Hepatol 2019;70(1):194–202.

31. Mantovani A, Dalbeni A. Treatments for NAFLD: State of Art. Int J Mol Sci 2021; 22(5):2350.

32. Polyzos SA, Kountouras J, Mantzoros CS. Obesity and nonalcoholic fatty liver disease: From pathophysiology to therapeutics. Metab Clin Exp 2019;92:82–97.

33. Matteoni CA, Younossi ZM, Gramlich T, et al. Nonalcoholic fatty liver disease: a spectrum of clinical and pathological severity. Gastroenterology 1999;116(6): 1413–9.

34. Hafeez S, Ahmed MH. Bariatric surgery as potential treatment for nonalcoholic fatty liver disease: a future treatment by choice or by chance? J Obes 2013; 2013:839275.

35. Aron-Wisnewsky J, Doré J, Clement K. The importance of the gut microbiota after bariatric surgery. Nat Rev Gastroenterol Hepatol 2012;9(10):590–8.

36. Cerreto M, Santopaolo F, Gasbarrini A, et al. Bariatric Surgery and Liver Disease: General Considerations and Role of the Gut-Liver Axis. Nutrients 2021;13(8): 2649.

37. Ruban A, Ashrafian H, Teare JP. The EndoBarrier: Duodenal-Jejunal Bypass Liner for Diabetes and Weight Loss. Gastroenterol Res Pract 2018;7823182.

Moving?

Make sure your subscription moves with you!

To notify us of your new address, find your **Clinics Account Number** (located on your mailing label above your name), and contact customer service at:

Email: journalscustomerservice-usa@elsevier.com

800-654-2452 (subscribers in the U.S. & Canada)
314-447-8871 (subscribers outside of the U.S. & Canada)

Fax number: 314-447-8029

Elsevier Health Sciences Division
Subscription Customer Service
3251 Riverport Lane
Maryland Heights, MO 63043

*To ensure uninterrupted delivery of your subscription, please notify us at least 4 weeks in advance of move.

Printed and bound by CPI Group (UK) Ltd, Croydon, CR0 4YY

08/05/2025

01864750-0007